Nursing Home Nightmares

Nursing Home Nightmares

Fighting for the Rights of Your Loved Ones

LAURA J. MULLINS
AND
WILLIAM G. PINTAS

EXPERT PRESS

Nursing Home Nightmares
Fighting for the Rights of Your Loved Ones

© 2019 Laura J. Mullins and William G. Pintas

ISBN-13: 978-1-946203-45-8

Pintas & Mullis Law Firm
368 W Huron St, Suite 100
Chicago, IL 60654
800-794-0444

.

Expert
Press

www.ExpertPress.net

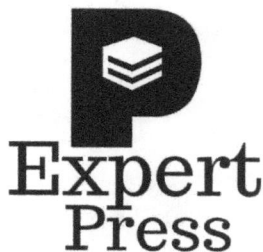

Contents

Introduction: A Loved One Is Going to a Nursing Home…   1

PART I: Finding a Good Nursing Home   7

Chapter 1: How to Know It's Time   9
Chapter 2: How to Pay for It   13
Chapter 3: How to Choose a Good Home   17

PART II: Injuries, Illness and More: What Can Go Wrong   23

Chapter 4: Common Types of Harm in the Nursing Home   25
Chapter 5: Other Types of Abuse and Injuries   35

PART III: What To Do If You Suspect Something Is Wrong   43

Chapter 6: Was This an Accident or Not?   45
Chapter 7: How Do You Know If Your Family Member Is
  Being Abused or Neglected?   55
Chapter 8: Changing Nursing Homes—How, When, and
  Why?   61

PART IV: How to Pursue Legal Action   67

Chapter 9: How Much Will It Cost? And Other Questions
  Answered   69
Chapter 10: Why Consider a Lawsuit?   79
Chapter 11: How and When Should I Hire a Lawyer?   85
Chapter 12: Now That You Have a Lawyer, What Should
  You Expect?   89
Chapter 13: Never Lose Faith—That's Why You Have a
  Lawyer   93

Conclusion: Why We Do What We Do   97

About the Authors   99

Introduction:

A Loved One Is Going to a Nursing Home…

WE KNOW THE EXTREME DIFFICULTY and often times gut-wrenching decisions families have to make before putting a loved one in a nursing home. Even though we are attorneys, we also have families and are faced with the very same difficult decisions. We wrote this book for our clients and their families.

In writing this book, we wanted to share with you the heartfelt truths along with the challenges we have seen after representing thousands of nursing home clients. We believe that, through our representation of residents and their families over the past thirty years, we have helped prompt some nursing homes to render better care.

Not all nursing homes are careless or neglectful. There are thousands of very hard-working and compassionate individuals working in nursing homes today. They are committed to quality care and treatment in this very difficult and challenging job. Unfortunately, most nursing homes are run for a profit and, as such, are underpaying, understaffing, and overworking their staff. Flawed ownership objectives will lead to poor management and, eventually, to poor care. This has been shown time and time again.

It is legal claims against this improper care that we hope will force nursing homes to operate as they promised you when you first brought your loved one to their home. Here is our story and experiences. We hope that this will shed some light on what to avoid so you and your loved ones will not fall victim to any nursing home nightmares.

In the beginning …

The very first nursing home case Pintas & Mullins ever took was perhaps our most memorable. It involved a 91-year-old former teacher named Susan Bell (whose name has been changed for the purposes of this book, as have all other names). Her sons were the ones who brought the case to our attention: three well-dressed, generally affable, middle-aged men, who were striking because of how worried and upset they were about their mother.

As they should have been, since Susan was suffering from horrific bedsores. Her nursing home, charged with providing her care and comfort, had allowed her condition to deteriorate appallingly. For ten years, she received good and caring support in that nursing home. However, once she was moved to a different floor of the nursing home, everything changed for the worse. After the move, Susan and her family began to suffer greatly. In a very short time, she began living, like so many before her, a nursing home nightmare.

Susan's sons came into our office, and we saw what we have seen so many times since: a family that is angry, scared, and most of all, confused and uncertain about what to do. The Bell family was generous at heart. One of the sons had donated a kidney in the recent past, and they all worked in community-focused jobs, like their mother before them. They just could not understand why this would happen to them and their mother.

Worse, they could not understand why no one would help. We were not the first attorneys they had spoken with. In fact, the Bell Family was told by another attorney that Susan was too old and too ill to proceed with a lawsuit.

When they came to us, the Bell sons wanted justice and better care for their mother, but at that point, they were feeling perhaps nothing could be done.

We have all heard nightmare stories like this before, stories of nursing homes providing criminally poor care, nursing homes that neglect and even abuse the elderly. Those stories are the first thing that come to mind when you discover that your loved one needs nursing home care.

We all want to believe "not me, not my family," but that denial can only get us so far. Nursing home neglect and abuse happens to families like yours and mine every day, all across the country. That insistence on denial often leaves families unprepared for the what may occur and filled with questions of what to do to protect their family in the event they do need a nursing home.

How do I find a place where these awful things won't happen to my loved one? How can I afford such a place? How do I balance location against reputation for a home? What do I do if an unthinkable nursing home nightmare does happen? How will I even know?

This book is designed to answer all of those questions and more. Our decades of experience have made it possible to provide this comprehensive guide that will help you to avoid what happened to Susan Bell, while also providing you with all the steps you need to take if the worst does happen.

The truth is, when it comes to nursing homes, what you don't know can lead to catastrophic events and injuries. Educating yourself will help you understand and take action in every potential situation.

In an ideal world, we would love to give you enough advice to guarantee your loved one will not suffer the way Susan Bell did, but we cannot do that. Unfortunately, cases of neglect and abuse in nursing homes are more prevalent than you think. What we can do is provide you with all the knowledge to take precautions while also preparing for the worst, so that, if that worst occurs, you can get the attention and justice you and your loved one deserve.

That's what we did for the Bell family. We took their case when others wouldn't, and we fought the nursing home hard for four years, through numerous difficulties. We fought through delays and misleading statements from the nursing home. We even fought through their bankruptcy to make sure Susan's family received the justice and compensation they deserved.

We started this book with the story of Susan Bell because we wanted to illustrate an important point: if the worst does happen to your loved one in a nursing home, you do not need to feel helpless. There are very strong laws to help and support you and your family in a nursing home claim. These laws help families get justice and compensation like they did the Bells, who saw their mother suffer instead of being cared for. These laws are written to protect the most vulnerable members of our society—our aging parents and grandparents—when they are unable to care and help themselves.

These nursing homes are often owned by large corporations who have spent their money on powerful lawyers instead of spending their money where it belongs, caring for our family members in need. These lawsuits do not just service victims and their families but also our community. It is important that nursing home owners know they cannot continue to neglect and abuse our loved ones. Everyone ages, regardless of your background or financial situation. Yet, almost no one imagines that they will become unable to care for themselves or their family members, leaving no choice but to move into a nursing home. The cases of neglect and abuse are, along with everything else, a gigantic violation of trust: to the individual, to the family, and to our whole society. It is our job to stand up and fight against that loss of trust and give families closure. It is important to know that there are resources that can help you change your loved one's conditions, resources that may get your family justice for what has already happened.

When incidents of neglect or abuse occur, many times we see that family members experience strong emotions of guilt for putting their loved one in the nursing home in the first place. They often blame themselves. The truth is, though, it is the nursing home's conduct that caused these injuries. Your lawyer's experience in nursing home cases is required since they will need to show and prove what happened.

This book provides a comprehensive guide to every part of the nursing home experience, so that, hopefully, you can avoid the nightmares if possible or handle them if they ever occur. We want to help the family with a loved one going into the nursing home; the family with concerns about a loved one already in the nursing home; and the family that knows something is wrong and needs to know what to do next.

Essentially, the purpose of this book is to guide you, step by step, from deciding when it is right to move a family member to a nursing home to when it is right to pursue a lawsuit on behalf of your family member.

Remember, the more prepared you are for the nursing home experience, the better chance you have of protecting your loved ones and avoiding ever needing to hire a lawyer.

We hope you find this guide helpful for you and your family.

PART I

FINDING A GOOD NURSING HOME

Chapter 1

How to Know It's Time

NO MATTER HOW your family member ends up in a nursing home, or when it happens in their lives, it is likely that you may feel a great deal of guilt about the event. Guilt is a significant factor in delaying the transition to the nursing home. It is also a huge barrier that keeps families from researching the details about when it is time to make that choice.

For many, they feel that they have somehow failed their loved one if they are no longer able to care for them at home. They feel they have let down those who cared for them when they were most vulnerable. They feel selfish and cruel.

These are all completely legitimate and natural feelings. However, someone growing old and ill is not your fault. Nursing home facilities are established for the sole purpose of caring for individuals in need. Almost no one at home can provide the kind of care needed for someone with serious failing health. People have jobs, children, and other responsibilities. Even when freed of those duties, caring for someone with degenerating health for 24 hours every day is simply impossible over any extended period.

Families across the country will experience these difficult decisions and feelings. Families should not feel guilty but should instead take some responsibility in choosing and visiting their family members residing in these long-term care facilities.

Although there is little that can be done to avoid sending a family member to a nursing home, there are a lot of other decisions and actions you can take to help your family member in need. We will discuss later in this chapter—and throughout the book—ways to help and hopefully avoid some nursing home nightmares.

We can all agree that nursing homes are necessary and serve a tremendous help in our country. Many good people work in nursing homes with the best of intentions, and much good work happens in many nursing homes. However, many bad things occur, too.

The better prepared you are for this responsibility, the easier it is to prepare for everything else in this book. Preparation now is key because, tragically, a lot of the time, the actual moment of transition to the nursing home is sudden. Most often an unexpected event will lead to the need for nursing home care.

With that in mind, we start this book by discussing how individuals end up in nursing homes. We hope this will help you prepare for when time it is right for your loved one.

There are four main ways somebody will require nursing home care, and most of them arise without warning.

The first reason for going to a nursing home is rehab. This is for a relatively short-term stay, usually for no more than a few months. Doctors may recommend rehab in a nursing home after an injury or an illness or following an extended hospital stay. Rehab will generally include physical therapy, speech therapy, or occupational therapy, among other options. The purpose and the goal of this nursing homestay is to get the resident stronger and back home. Unfortunately, many times that does not happen.

While rehab is designed to be short-term, it is important to point out that it does not always work out that way. If the resident is unable get their strength back and rehab is unsuccessful, your loved one may be transitioned into long-term care (more about which below). Also of note, while the rehab may be planned, most hospital stays are unexpected. Thereby, a nursing home stay may sneak up on a family.

The second reason that somebody goes to a nursing home is probably the one most people think about: long-term care. This is for those who have no real likelihood of getting rehabbed and require

24-hour care. In the long-term scenario, your family member may enter the nursing home either straight from their home or from the hospital.

When a family member enters the nursing home from their family home, it is commonly because of deterioration in their condition, often dementia or Alzheimer's. As the disease progresses, your loved one becomes more difficult to care for at home. At some point, the amount of care required becomes too much for a family to take on. A loved one with dementia may get worse at night and start wandering, leaving the house when everyone is asleep. This and other forms of deterioration can be unsafe for the individual and for the family. In that situation, a doctor will likely recommend moving your loved one to a nursing home.

From the hospital, there are two common scenarios that can play out. The first involves a hospitalization due to a catastrophic event, leaving the family with little or no hope of recovery. A common example of this is a very massive stroke that leaves the individual immobile and possibly non-verbal. The other situation is the one mentioned above, when somebody becomes a long-term care resident after they were initially sent for rehab.

The third way a family member can enter the nursing home is a transition from assisted living to long-term nursing home care. Assisted living is an in-between residence where some assistance is provided but your family member remains fairly self-sufficient. This is ideal for those who just need some regular but not constant help.

Over time, however, as their health declines, the assisted living facility may no longer feel capable of handling your family member's needs. This often occurs when they become less mobile, which means your loved one's care becomes more of a 24/7 requirement instead of a part of regular (but not constant) attendance. In that situation, the assisted living facility should recommend moving your loved one over to a skilled nursing home for long-term admission.

The final and least common situation that results in nursing home care is what is called "respite care." This is a short-term option for those who are caring for their loved one at home. For anyone who has cared for or still cares for a loved one in poor health, they know this is a full-time job, even with home health support. As a full-time caretaker who is unable to get away without harming the health and comfort of your loved one, you obviously get worn down. You need a break. Whether it's a day off or a proper vacation, or dealing with your own medical needs, you need a chance to rest and take care of yourself.

Nursing homes provide "respite" care that is usually just for a month or less. In this situation, unlike the others above, you usually have time to prepare and find a home and situation that is appropriate for you and your loved one's needs.

A somewhat unrelated way some individuals enter the nursing home is through mental illness and homelessness. They are placed in long-term care because they need consistent looking after and have nowhere else to go. Certain homes may be more commonly used for mental illness and homelessness. Those generally have slightly younger residents. Be sure to ask your prospective nursing homes about this if you feel it is a concern.

No matter the reason your loved one ends up needing nursing home care, you have to remember that this is, to some extent, an inevitable process. At such a moment, it is important to recognize that you are not failing your loved one. After all, this is why nursing homes exist. However, when that moment comes, it is important to recognize that your responsibilities for your loved one have not ended, they have just changed.

As we will discuss in later chapters, your role transforms from one of immediate care to overall watchfulness. You will need to find the right home and make sure that the home is taking care of your loved one. If something goes wrong, you then need to find someone to get justice for them.

Chapter 2

How to Pay for It

ONE OF THE MAJOR CONCERNS about nursing home care is always the cost. When the need to place a loved one in the nursing home suddenly arises, there can be a moment of panic not just over their personal well-being but also over the family finances.

For those who qualify for state benefits, paying for a nursing home will not financially damage a family. In that case, it is actually one of the more straightforward parts of the nursing home process, one that your nursing home will help you work through.

However, for others, the process can be much more complex. It is important to speak to nursing homes up front and find out what kind of financial burden will be placed upon your loved one and upon you.

Often, the nursing home will work with you to help place your loved one on state benefits, but be sure to pay attention to what you are signing. Ask questions and seek assistance to ensure you fully understand all of the admission documents and financial responsibility.

Whether paid for outright or through state Medicaid funds, paying for a nursing home can occur in several different ways, all dependent upon the age and financial situation of the admitted resident.

To begin with, the vast majority of those entering a nursing home are over the age of 65, and are therefore Medicare eligible. This is important because although Medicare will not pay for long-term care, it usually covers nursing home rehab. Medicare will pay for 100 days of rehab. Once those 100 days of rehab are up, though, the family will have some harder choices if their loved one is not progressing as anticipated. At that point, any further rehab would be out of pocket. Otherwise, they become long-term patients.

In long-term care, Medicaid usually steps in and covers the payments. For those elderly individuals who already have limited funds, this is, once again, very straightforward. Otherwise, a loved one must become "Medicaid eligible." If your loved one has too much money to qualify for Medicaid but not enough to pay for their long-term stay, most nursing homes will help them reorganize their finances and complete the paperwork so they can apply for Medicaid. At that point, they would become what's called "Medicaid pending." However, part of this process would usually require your family member entering the nursing home to turn over their social security and other income to the home.

Regardless, the individual either on Medicaid or becoming Medicaid eligible will have to find a nursing home with a "Medicaid bed." These are different than private beds, which are more readily available for those who have the (significant) funds to cover the stay privately.

Each nursing home will have a certain, limited number of Medicaid beds. So, it is important to find a nursing home that has one-such bed available if you need immediate entry. When no beds are available, the applicant is placed on a waitlist. This can either be a short delay or can take a significant amount of time. It can even take years in some cases.

The only way to avoid this situation entirely is to either have the funds to pay for the stay outright, or in a somewhat rarer option, to pay for the stay through a long-term care insurance policy. While rare, this can work to the individual's advantage, since long-term care insurance can provide access to private beds, making it easier to get admitted anywhere the family prefers.

For the majority of people who lack either the means or the insurance to get a private bed, this is an important moment to be vigilant in the nursing home process. While it is nice that nursing homes provide a service in helping families get through all that paperwork, do not simply trust them to settle the finances to your best possible interest. Read every document you sign carefully. For example, avoid signing any document that contains an "arbitration clause." A lot of nursing homes try to sneak these in with other paperwork. If you and/or your loved one sign that, it may limit your legal options if anything goes wrong.

A second major concern, if you have power of attorney for your relative, is to make sure you are not taking personal responsibility for any of the billing outside of your duties as power of attorney. This is a complicated issue that does not need to be worked through here, but be sure to ask the nursing home to make sure you are not personally responsible for any costs.

To summarize all of the above, the good news is that nursing home care does not have to cost you and your loved one anything beyond what they already have (in savings, social security, etc.), unless you are able to pay for a private bed. While it may take several different roads to reach the final payment method, nursing home care will be available to your loved one without bankrupting your whole family.

Still, it is best to be careful and find the best way to cover the nursing home while not signing away any rights or income the nursing home has no right to demand.

Chapter 3

How to Choose a Good Home

UNFORTUNATELY, WE NEED TO STATE two uncomfortable and unfortunate points up front in this chapter. First, there is no guarantee that the nursing home you choose for your loved one will be free of instances of abuse or neglect. Second, there is no guarantee that even a good nursing home will remain good.

If you remember the story of Susan Bell in the introduction, she spent 10 successful and happy years at her nursing home before her care suddenly went downhill. In her case, it was a matter of being moved to a different floor where the care was not as high quality, but it can just as easily be a change in management or personnel that leads to a decrease in the quality of care.

Beyond those two points, it is also often the case that bad things happen in the "good homes" that are otherwise well run, while good things happen in the homes with a reputation as "bad homes."

The stubborn and frustrating fact is that you just cannot simply choose a home and trust in the care. That is precisely the reason you must continue to always remain vigilant for your loved one and maintain access all the tools you need to avoid neglect and abuse.

All that being said, you must always do research to find the best possible nursing home for your loved one upfront. There are certainly better run and worse run homes, and the better the home your family member enters, the better their chance of avoiding any negative and catastrophic experiences.

To figure out which nursing home is best for you, we recommend visiting all the homes you are considering before making a decision. Find all the homes that have availability and physically set foot in each of them.

When visiting, it is important to use all of your senses. Begin with sight: What do you see? Do you see residents looking clean and happy? Do you see staff members actively working and engaging with the residents? Or, do you see them sitting around at the desk and doing nothing? Does the place look clean, or does it look filthy? Is it well-lit or dark?

Now, take in all the smells. This is one of the most important senses to use upon entering a nursing home. Take a basic sniff test and decide if the facility smells clean or like urine. We have spoken to a lot of families that say as soon as they walked into a particular home, they knew something was going wrong simply because of the smell.

Next, make a mental note of the sounds you hear. Are you hearing call alarms going off without nurses attending to the residents? Are residents yelling out for help or attention and not being answered? Listen for the sounds of different activities being performed. Listen for calm voices or shouting. At the same time, listen for laughter and good humor. The presence or absence of these sounds give you a general sense of an environment. Essentially, does the nursing home you are entering sound like an environment where everyone seems to be happy and comfortable or like a very sterile and cold place?

The final sense you should use isn't quite the one you would expect. While it's good to use your sense of touch as well (and taste if you can sample the food), the one you really should concentrate on is your gut feeling. As soon as you walk in, you will have an instinctive reaction. We tell everyone who asks for our advice the same thing on this topic: "Use your instinct. It is almost always accurate." Using all your senses helps create a solid sense of whether a nursing home is right for your family, and using your gut feeling will tell you more than any other sense. Trust it.

There is second major factor to consider when finding a nursing home: the location. In many ways, this is just as important, sometimes even more important, than your general impression of the home itself.

As will be discussed more in later chapters, perhaps the single best thing you can do to protect your relative from a nursing home nightmare is to visit often and to visit at different times and on different days. Nursing homes often make a mental note of the schedules of visiting family. If you visit at the same time every day or every week, they know to get your family member cleaned up and looking good for that hour. If you only ever visit for that hour, you do not truly know how your family member is doing during the other 167 hours a week.

Having the ability to pop in at different times of the day is a gigantic benefit to your family member. First of all, it has a profoundly beneficial aspect to their quality of life, knowing they will see family regularly. But just as important is your ability to make sure you are getting the best care for your loved one every hour of the day and every day of the week.

The last thing we recommend when looking for a nursing home is to check the reviews and ratings. This is far easier than in the past, since there are now plenty of online resources to check.

To begin with, each state should have a website listing all of their nursing homes. These sites also keep track of complaints that were filed by family members. Now, it is important to recognize that every nursing home is going to have at least a few complaints filed against them, so don't rule out one just because a complaint was issued.

Instead, we recommend looking at the quantity of complaints filed by family members to assess any patterns of neglect and mistreatment. That is a much more effective test than whether any violations were found or not. Finding a home with only two or three complaints over the past year would be an indicator of a better nursing home compared to a nursing home that received six or seven complaints over the past month.

Even if those seven complaints at the one home were found as unfounded or no violation, it still means that family members were not happy with the care received and upset enough to take the effort to contact the state and file the complaint.

Beyond the state websites, Medicare (https://www.medicare.gov/nursinghomecompare/search.html) and U.S. Health and News (https://health.usnews.com/best-nursing-homes) offer rankings and reviews of nursing homes. These can also be an extremely beneficial ways to find out the standing and rating of the nursing home you are considering.

Once you have a nursing home that has passed the sense test, is in a reasonable location for your family, and has reviews you can live with, one final consideration may affect your nursing home decision. It relates to the specific care needs of your family member. If your family member has a tracheotomy, you should make sure that the nursing home has the facilities and experience to specifically handle those needs. If your loved one has a significant wound that requires regular wound care, ask the nursing home if it has the ability handle that kind of care.

This may or may not be a major focus in the case of your family member, but it is always good to ask nursing home representatives about the staff's experience in handling these medical conditions.

This can be a matter of life and death in some cases. Susan Bell may not have developed severe bedsores if her nursing home had enough staff that was capable of providing advanced Alzheimer's care.

It would be nice if Susan's story was rare, but it isn't. Another client of ours was the sister of a woman named Heather Reed. Heather was 72 years old, blind, bedridden, and on dialysis when she was admitted to her nursing home.

Unfortunately, because her need for a nursing home came unexpectedly after she suffered a massive heart attack, her sister Mary didn't have time to find a home that had on-site dialysis.

Initially, this was not a problem. However, one Tuesday, Mary got a call from her sister complaining that she wasn't feeling very well. It turned out that the nursing home failed to take Heather for dialysis. It had been three days since her last session.

The next day Mary called the nursing home to check on the situation, at which point, she found out that her sister still had not been sent out for dialysis. Mary rushed to the nursing home the next day and demanded to know why she was not sent out for her needed dialysis. The nursing home casually informed her that the transportation company they used to send patients out on dialysis had been absent for much of the past week.

Mary's frustration at this situation quickly turned to tragedy. While Mary was panicking over the nursing home's failure to provide the necessary transportation, Heather suddenly passed out. She was rushed to the hospital, but there was little they could do at that point. She died that same day. Mary requested an autopsy, and it came back with the expected results: kidney failure and heart failure because Heather had gone five days without dialysis.

Mary retained our office. A lawsuit was filed against the nursing home and the transportation company. After several years of litigation, we brought closure for Mary along with a substantial settlement.

While not everyone's case ends as tragically as Heather's, her and Susan's stories are warnings of what can happen if a nursing home is not equipped to handle the specific needs of its residents.

And that warning extends to all advice in this chapter. These tragic outcomes can occur anywhere, but the more prepared you are to find the best possible home and to visit as often as possible, the better chance your loved one will not suffer neglect like Heather and Susan suffered.

PART II

Injuries, Illness, and More:
What Can Go Wrong

Chapter 4

Common Types of Harm

in the Nursing Home

AS WE HAVE ALREADY MENTIONED several times in this book, once your loved one is in a nursing home, your care and responsibility for them does not end, it simply changes. At this point, it is now time to focus on watching out for their well-being within the nursing home environment and making sure they are getting the care and attention they need every day.

The best way to help your loved one is to remain active in their lives, visiting regularly and remaining in regular contact with the nursing home. Part of that new focus on vigilance is the need to be aware of what kind of harm can come from nursing home neglect and abuse so you can see the warning signs and know when to react.

This and the next two chapters will cover a lot of tragic and tragically common forms of injury and harm that can occur to those in nursing homes. To begin, we will cover the three most common threats to your loved one's health and wellbeing once they enter a home: bedsores, falls, and infection.

Bedsores

A bedsore is one of the most common reasons for filing lawsuits. Bedsores, also known as pressure injury or decubitus ulcers, are very painful, dangerous, and commonly caused by neglect.

In one example, our office represented the family of Martina Costa, an Italian-born 79-year-old who was suffering from Parkinson's disease. Despite that fact, she was doing pretty well and living at home until she required hospitalization for a couple of weeks on an unrelated issue. The hospital recommended rehab for her, and she was therefore released to a nursing home for an anticipated short duration.

Her family helped her choose her first nursing home based off her language limitations. Martina only spoke Italian, and the family was thrilled to find a local nursing home with Italian speaking staff members. However, they soon realized they were not happy with the quality of care at that facility, and so, after a short period, moved her to a different nursing home.

This is where the story took something of a twist. After Martina arrived at her second home, the second facility reported a bedsore, which the family assumed at the time started and developed at the first facility. That was a reasonable assumption, of course, because the family had a lot of complaints about the lack of quality care that she had been receiving.

The family contacted our office to investigate a case against the first nursing home due to the development of a horrific bedsore. Once we got involved and obtained and reviewed all of the necessary medical records, we discovered that the horrific bedsore was actually due to neglect at the second nursing home.

When Martina was admitted to the second nursing home, all she had was a very minor skin breakdown, something any caring and attentive nursing home should have been able to handle and heal. It only took two weeks of poor care from the second home for that minor issue to progress into a deep and infected stage 4 bedsore. Although she went through several surgeries, her bedsore never healed, and Martina ended up dying from the wound.

We mention Martina Costa because her case, just like Susan Bell's, so clearly illustrates how dangerous bedsores are and also how hard it is to remain on top of the quality of care your loved one is receiving. These cases show why it is important to know as much about bedsores as you can, so that you know how to recognize them immediately and do something about them before they become too serious to heal.

With that point in mind, what exactly are bedsores? Bedsores are the results of too much pressure on a particular point. When somebody is not moved enough, and the skin has too much pressure on it in one position, it can cause a breakdown in the skin tissue that then leads to severe skin injuries. They are normally found on the parts of the body that experience this pressure while laying down. Bedsores are often found, in particular, around the tailbone, buttocks, and the hips, but they aren't limited to those areas. They can also appear in such areas as the heel, the ear, and the shoulder, among others.

The pressure part of bedsores is why they are also called pressure wounds, although a more precise (and these days preferred) term is "pressure injury." The National Pressure Ulcer Advisory Panel has recently made this exact change because "injury" better shows that bedsores are preventable.

This idea of preventability helps us arrive at the most essential fact about bedsores: they can, for the most part, be avoided with the right care. If a patient is getting enough nutrients in their diet, and if they are turning and repositioning (or being turned and repositioned) enough, they should not develop pressure injuries.

Bedsores, as you might expect, mostly develop when someone is elderly and immobile. In other words, when their bodies struggle to heal and they are unable to turn themselves regularly, bedsores become more likely. In that case, the protocol to prevent pressure injuries or bedsores is to turn and reposition the resident every 2 hours, 24 hours a day. If that regimen is kept up, the person likely should not develop bedsores. However, when somebody who is not able to turn or move on their own and is not being turned and repositioned by their caretakers at such regular intervals, those pressure points can lead to bedsores stunningly quickly.

When a pressure injury starts, they are rated, or "staged," from one to four. A stage 1 injury would show a reddening of the skin.

If dealt with properly at that point, it should be able to heal pretty quickly. A stage 2 injury looks kind of like a burn mark, where a couple layers of the skin are gone. A stage 3 injury is an open wound. It's deep, and it goes into the muscle. A stage 4 pressure injury is the highest and most severe stage. It is an open wound that is so deep that the bone is now exposed.

Bedsores at any stage can get better under the right circumstances and if the patient is healthy and strong enough, but they don't always. Even when they do heal, it can take quite a bit of time. If a bedsore reaches stage 4, for instance, it can take months—sometimes a year or two—to heal fully. Even then, it can leave scarring and continue to cause pain.

The best way to make sure your loved one avoids bedsores is to pay attention to their risk factors and their diet. Any mention that your loved one is at risk of bedsores should be met with great concern on your part, and on the part of the nursing home. Your loved one's nursing home should develop a care plan that helps avoid this risk.

This is very important because, bedsores are one of the most common nursing home catastrophes. Once a bedsore develops, it can increase in size and seriousness horrifyingly quickly, and the end result is too often death.

Falls

The second most common nursing home injury that brings family members to our office is the result of a fall. It is important to note that many falls in a nursing home are, like bedsores, mostly preventable. That is, after all, one of the main reasons we send our loved ones to a nursing home: to protect them from such events. Very often, they are sent to the nursing to recover from a fall at home

Most of our clients who have been injured as a result of a fall at the nursing home had prior fall incidents. This means, upon the admission to the nursing home or perhaps during the duration of the nursing home stay, these residents were noted or should have been noted as a fall risk. Once deemed at risk for falls, the nursing home must prepare a care plan in an attempt to prevent falls and injuries. This is one of the most crucial parts of nursing home care because, after all, it is impossible to watch someone 24 hours a day, 7 days a week. To keep your loved one safe, the nursing home needs an individualized care plan to reduce the risk of falls and the risk of injury should a fall occur.

Some factors that lead to a higher risk of fall are: an unsteady gait, rehab needs, and dementia or Alzheimer's. In that final case, the resident is no longer able to comprehend that they can no longer walk or are no longer as strong as they were, so they continue to try to get up on their own.

For those who are at risk (or, of course, even occasionally those who are not), a fall can occur anywhere in the nursing home. For unsteady walkers, a small spill, uneven carpet, or some debris that hasn't been cleaned up can be enough to cause a fall. For those who are mostly immobile, falling out of bed or out of a wheelchair is common. We also see many falls—or, more accurately, drops—due directly to the nursing staff, especially during a transfer from bed to wheelchair or wheelchair to bed. If a resident is assessed as needing a two-person assist when being moved, and the nursing home is understaffed, we commonly see injuries occur when only one person handles the transfer.

Falls are also often related to the very tools that are meant to help those who struggle to move. Many residents fall because their wheelchair or walker has been placed or moved away from the bed or resident. That means the resident is required to try to get up to reach their wheelchair or the walker, at which point they are at high risk of falling. Other examples include when the nursing home fails to lock the wheels on the wheelchair or bed. When the resident reaches for support, the bed or wheelchair move.

This example brings us to an important point: as a general rule, if your loved one requires assistance with mobility, such as a wheelchair, there's almost always a risk of falling. If that statement applies to your loved one, there are a couple things that you can do to help prevent falls. One is putting a wedge between their legs, like a pillow. That would help people who have a tendency to slump forward, preventing them from sliding out of the wheelchair.

Another option is what is called a lap-buddy, which is like a seat belt. However, while that might sound like an ideal option for the wheelchair, many states have laws against restraining individuals, and those wheelchair seat belts can count as a restraint. There are also bed rails to prevent patients getting out of bed to reach their wheelchair or walking device or falling out while sleeping. However, once again, that option often goes against the same restraint laws, and many times, a doctor's order is required. You will need to consult your nursing home about how you can implement those options.

Even without any form of restraint, though, nursing homes can still do a lot. Bed and chair alarms are available to help alert the nursing staff if a high-risk resident has gotten out of bed or the wheelchair. Although these devices may not prevent all falls, they certainly can notify the staff to act quickly and possibly prevent a fall. Other options that may not prevent all falls but can greatly reduce the risk of injury from a fall include moving the bed low to the ground; placing mats next to bed; and ensuring the call button is always within reach. All together, these tools, when implemented properly, can significantly reduce the risk and severity of falls.

Unfortunately, when falls do occur, serious injuries are very often the result. The most common injury is perhaps the most famous: the broken hip. After that, the second most common is a head injury, in particular bleeding in the brain. Less serious injuries might include bruising, black eyes, and cuts and lacerations that require stitches.

For those who are particularly concerned about the risk of a fall for their loved one, there is a final option available to families who can afford it. That option is to hire a private sitter who stays with your loved one throughout the day to make sure they are well cared for and safe. The benefits of this are obvious, particularly when it comes to the risk of falls. However, even those families with private sitters still face the risk of their loved ones falling.

We once had a case that involved a family with a very good private sitter for their father, whose name was Jerry Swift. However, the sitter still needed some time off to live his own life, and the family had agreed to give Sunday's off. On one such Sunday, the family called to check on Jerry, and the nursing home told them that he was in the dining room in his wheelchair.

The family assumed everything was fine, but when they called just a little later, they found out that a custodian in the building had found Jerry at the bottom of a staircase with his wheelchair on top of him. The nursing home was unable to tell the family how long he had been there. Our investigation uncovered that somebody in the nursing home had left the door down to the laundry open, and Jerry, who had dementia, thought by going through the door he might get out of the nursing home. He got out of the dining room without being noticed, went through the open door, and ended up with a tragic ending.

Jerry was immediately hospitalized with a broken eye socket and a brain bleed. He was unable to breathe on his own and placed on a ventilator. Due to the severity of his injuries, Jerry died three months later. This tragic story, like many others we have represented, was completely avoidable.

Jerry's case really highlights just how difficult it is to avoid these risks even when you are vigilant. The Swift family did everything right, and still, somehow, Jerry ended up suffering a fatal injury.

Infections

Our final category in this chapter is infections. Infections, like bedsores and falls, are really common and really dangerous in nursing homes. When you have a lot of elderly people with different health conditions in a confined space, infections will be found.

Perhaps the most common infection is the urinary tract infection, commonly referred to as a UTI. While UTIs are relatively common in normal life as well, they are much more common and much more complicated in the nursing home setting. To begin with, they are somewhat unavoidable with all the use of catheters, and this is exacerbated by many nursing homes leaving catheters in longer than necessary, out of convenience.

While many might only associated UTIs with mild discomfort, in a nursing home, they are much more serious. If a UTI is not diagnosed in a timely manner or is undiagnosed and progresses, it can become really dangerous and fatal. The infection can reach the bloodstream and the resident can quickly become septic. A further complication in the nursing home is that many residents are unable to communicate that they are suffering from the signs and symptoms of a UTI. These residents are simply not able to complain of painful urination, having frequent urination, or a foul odor.

If the nursing home staff are not attentive, the signs of a severe infection can easily be missed, allowing the infection to progress and become dangerous.

This can become a chronic problem for nursing home residents. One of our previous clients, a woman named Josephine Sanders, went through five years of chronic UTIs. She would develop them every month for years.

Her family called us wondering if something was wrong, but proving infections are due to poor care is not always simple. We took the case. During this time Josephine's family moved her to another nursing home, where she received much better care. As soon as she got to the new nursing home, amazingly, Josephine went an entire year without ever going to the hospital for an infection.

Such a night and day difference demonstrated just how important good and hygienic nursing home care can be to avoiding infection. Whether it's a lack of proper staffing or a lack of proper hygiene, a nursing home may not be able to avoid all infection, but they can cause more of it.

Thankfully, Josephine got out of that home when she did, and she lived several years on afterward in a home where she was much more comfortable.

Another common infection in nursing homes is *Clostridium difficile*, or C-diff. C-diff usually develops after a high use of antibiotics. It results in diarrhea, which can lead to dehydration and kidney failure. This can be fatal, particularly to the elderly.

Often times, C-diff is unavoidable for the elderly simply because they have to be on antibiotics so often. However, C-diff is also highly contagious, and therefore, the nursing home can be responsible for spreading it due to poor hygiene. This leads to residents who are not generally at risk developing C-diff. Often, these residents are not on antibiotics, but their roommate is. Alternatively, the nursing staff is treating another resident with C-diff and do not properly wash their hands. When a resident is under treatment for C-diff infection, they should be isolated from the other residents to prevent the spread of this serious infection.

Because of how easy it is to spread and how long it takes to treat (several months), it's very common for it to spread through an entire nursing home due to poor care by the nursing staff.

Another risky infection in nursing homes is the antibiotic resistant MRSA super bug. MRSA is especially common in hospital and nursing home settings. It usually enters through the skin, often through an open wound, and it then gets into the bloodstream.

The final common infection is perhaps the most famous: pneumonia. This is a lung infection, and similar to the other infections, it is somewhat unavoidable in a nursing home. However, if your loved one is regularly getting pneumonia (and/or different infections) it's something to definitely be concerned about.

That last point is worth emphasizing: any time your family member contracts an infection, it should be cause for concern, and if they are regularly contracting infections, or falling, or showing signs of bedsores, it is time to consider whether you should be taking more significant steps (which we will discuss in later chapters).

All of these issues can, to a greater or lesser degree, occur naturally in a nursing home environment. However, the nursing home can undeniably exacerbate or even cause all of these issues. Proper care plans that are followed thoroughly, enough staff to handle resident needs, and the overall hygiene and cleanliness of the nursing home are all important factors in the likelihood your loved one will be at a greater or lesser risk for any of the above mentioned situations.

Chapter 5

Other Types of Abuse and Injuries

IT IS AN UNFORTUNATE FACT that the risks found in a nursing home do not end with those listed in the last chapter. In fact, in some ways, they can get much worse. All of the previously mentioned risks are in some way natural. Those who are immobile are prone to bedsores, those who struggle to walk can fall, and living in close quarters with many others raises the risk of infection. While nursing homes can and should do more to avoid all these issues, they are not usually intentionally done. However, that is not always the case.

Some incidents are committed through choices made in the nursing home, whether those be criminal acts by the staff or the choice by managers to remain understaffed. This chapter will briefly cover many of the nightmares that can grow out of these intentional actions.

Physical Assault

Physical assault, in one form or another, is more common in a nursing home setting than many realize. We often see injuries from physical assault, with the most common form coming from resident-on-resident attacks. This is often a situation in which one resident has dementia, schizophrenia, or some other mental health issues, and this individual suddenly attacks another resident.

Or, it may seem sudden, from outside. The reality is that the nursing home is most likely aware of those residents with such behavior or tendencies. These residents need to be handled carefully and closely monitored, but often are not. In fact, very often, these known aggressors are mixed in with all the other residents without any extra attention or monitoring until something awful happens.

Assaults are not just from aggressive residents, but often from the very people hired to take care of our loved ones. There is plenty of rough handling by the nursing staff as well. We have represented many families concerning injuries that occurred due to rough care from nurses when turning, bathing, carrying, or otherwise caring for residents. This roughness leads to significant bruising, as well as feelings of fear, worry, and sometimes, depression.

It is important to watch out for mysterious bruising or changes in personality that might suggest a physical assault is taking place. Many residents, even when they are able, do not directly communicate these issues, so be extra vigilant.

Sexual Assault

That same warning about extra vigilance also applies to sexual assaults. If anything, sexual assaults are reported even less often than physical assaults, but that does not mean they are not just as tragically common.

We find that the assailants are not the nursing home staff but, often times, are other residents or even visitors to the nursing home. We have seen numerous instances in which a resident begins a sexual relationship with another resident who is incapable of consenting. They simply no longer have the mental capacity to make that decision. It is the nursing home's job to protect such residents, but again, they often fail to do so.

That is only the beginning of how nursing homes can fall short on this issue. There are plenty of cases—some of them quite famous—of nursing home staff assaulting residents. This can occur to men or women, at any age, either competent or not competent to consent. In short, it can happen to anyone in a nursing home.

One of our previous cases involved just such an incident. Janet Peters was mentally competent and in generally good health. She was still living on her own (her husband had just recently died) and was admitted to the nursing home for rehab after a hip injury. During Janet's short stay of just a few months, a male nurse began giving her a suspicious amount of attention. Others noticed this, but no one made any effort to investigate.

Because no one stepped in, this male nurse took advantage of Janet and started giving her showers, despite the fact that she had repeatedly requested a female assistant. He then began touching her inappropriately during these showers. This continued over a period of weeks and progressively got worse. He even invited others to engage in similar behavior. Eventually, he forced her to perform oral sex on him.

Janet was terrified and afraid to say anything, even after she got home. In fact, she only said something when her son noticed a dramatic change in her behavior. She was a lively and chipper person before the nursing home but had since become depressed. If it had not been for his concern, this nurse may have gotten away with these horrendous actions and even tried them again.

Thankfully, Janet's son finally got the story out, the police were immediately notified, and the nurse was arrested and charged. We successfully held the nursing home responsible for this horrific action.

Food- and Drink-Related Issues

With nursing homes, not every issue that causes harm is so grossly intentional. For example, many food and drink related issues can simply be related to a lack of staff and time.

There are, for instance, many choking and dehydration risks in nursing homes that do not develop out of any malice or intentionally poor care, only out of sloppiness, understaffing, and a lack of focus on individual patient needs.

For instance, our firm represented the family of a 63-year-old schizophrenic woman named Naomi Pitt. Naomi had been living successfully on her own, but as her mental abilities began to decline significantly, her family admitted her into a nursing home for long-term care, where she stayed for two years.

When the family came to visit one time, they noticed that she was having difficulty eating and swallowing. The doctors gave her a swallow evaluation to test her risk factors, and it came back showing that she needed to be on a puree diet with no solid foods. The nursing home complied to the doctor's recommendations and kept Naomi on a puree diet that removed any choking hazard.

However, a couple months after the diagnosis, a nurse was delivering meals on a food cart. They were going through the hallways with a pile of sandwiches on the cart and regularly stepping away, leaving the cart and the food completely unattended. During one of these moments, Naomi ran to the cart, grabbed a couple sandwiches, and ran back to her room to eat these sandwiches. Tragically, this seemingly innocent behavior of sneaking some sandwiches turned deadly. Naomi, unable to comprehend her swallowing limitations, began choking and passed out. The nurses found her and performed CPR for almost 40 minutes, but because of the loss of oxygen, she never recovered.

That story really shows just how important the role of every staff member in the nursing home is, and how important it is for nursing homes to have enough staff to remain focused. One nurse losing focus and forgetting about a resident's specific care plan led to a fatal outcome.

A similar issue involving focus and staffing is dehydration. To illustrate this, it's best to relay another story from one of our clients. Michael Kemper was a joyful man, even as Parkinson's and dementia began to limit his movements. He remained invested in his life, but he struggled with eating and drinking on his own and required assistance during meal times. The nursing home needed an aid to help feed him and make sure he was drinking enough water, but unfortunately, this nursing home, like most nursing homes, was grossly understaffed.

So, while he received all of his meals, he was not given any assistance and, therefore, couldn't consume the meals. Worse, food trays were often placed at a distance where he could not easily reach. While Michael's family tried to communicate this problem, the nursing home neither took note nor action. They also did not seem to care that his collected food trays were still full of food and water, documenting how little Michael was consuming. These careless mistakes on the nursing home's part led to severe dehydration for Michael that almost led to kidney failure. Thankfully, his family discovered what was happening in time, and Michael made a full recovery.

As Michael's case illustrates, fortunately, a dehydration diagnosis caught early is treatable, and most residents can get rehydrated with minimal damage. That all depends on how quickly the issue is spotted, though, and nursing homes that fail to notice what food is not being eaten are not likely to notice the signs of dehydration, such as a sudden loss of weight.

Michael's story also shows that often meal time is rushed in the nursing home, and many elderly struggle to eat and drink quickly. The residents need assistance with every bite and every sip. This is time-consuming work, and understaffed nursing homes simply do not have the people and time to care for the required needs of our family members. Cutting meals short can lead to severe and serious malnutrition and dehydration issues. This, in turn, can lead to kidney failure and death.

Theft

When it comes to personal items, the simple truth is: do not expect to see these items again if you leave them in a nursing home. That's how prevalent theft is in the nursing home environment. To begin with, clothing that family members leave for residents almost always gets recycled into the general nursing home supply. The laundry in the nursing home is not done individually; it all gets mixed together. It is likely you may find your loved one's clothing on another resident. That is assuming you ever see it again at all. If the means and time are available, you may want to take your loved one's laundry home to care for it.

On some level, such theft can perhaps be justified by the needs and limitations of the nursing home, but that does not mean it is not theft. It is justifiably upsetting. Even more upsetting, and far, far worse, are more direct and purposeful acts of theft.

The most traumatic theft story our firm has dealt with involved a man collecting the belongings of his mother, Sarah Jones, after she passed. During the process of bringing in the coroner and making funeral arrangements, the man stepped away from Sarah's remains very briefly. In that time, one of the staff members of the nursing home entered the room and stole her jewelry right off her body. Sarah's son immediately called the police and thankfully the jewelry was recovered, but it was a traumatic experience at a moment that was already incredibly difficult. Not every case ends so neatly. Many family members experience the same issue but are not in the frame of mind to notice a missing ring or necklace. By the time they do, it may be too late.

However, while such extreme cases are by no means rare, the majority of the theft that takes place in a nursing home is closer to the clothing example than the jewelry example. Objects like sweaters and shoes are almost certain to disappear over time in a nursing home. As a general rule, it is best to assume any object you leave with your loved one in a nursing home has a high probability of being lost or stolen during your loved one's time there. So, plan accordingly.

Neglect and Poor Care

"Neglect and Poor Care" is a very broad category, and one that could very much describe many of the issues covered in this book. In this section, though, it is best to think of those terms as relating to shortcuts nursing home staff take in order to make their jobs easier or to accommodate understaffing, even when it is unhealthy, unsafe, or degrading to their residents.

One of the big issues in this category is overmedication. You may suddenly notice that your family member is sleeping all of the time or seems groggy at all hours. If so, it is time to check and see if there's been a medication change. We find, a lot of times, especially with dementia residents, that nurses overmedicate just to remove some of their responsibilities of care. We call this "medical restraint" or "chemical restraint."

Obviously, it is much easier to care for somebody sleeping than it is to chase somebody who's active and screaming. Dementia patients may cause a certain amount of havoc in a nursing home—they may, for instance, be responsible for the physical abuse mentioned above—and they require that extra level of supervision and care because of it. The quickest and easiest way to handle somebody like that is not the healthy, safe, and optimal way a resident or their family would prefer. Instead, the easiest thing to do is to overmedicate them. Then, they are in bed all the time and a problem for no one.

For the nurse, that sounds ideal, but for the resident, it raises the risk factors that can lead to a decline in health or other physical injuries.

Beyond overmedication, nursing homes also often use bedpans and diapers for those residents who are still continent. Even though they are able to control themselves, it is simply easier for the nursing staff to use these humiliating methods to decrease their workload. Using diapers and bedpans places a resident on the nurses' schedule, instead of the other way around. It makes it possible for them to ignore the call light for trips to the bathroom.

This lack of response to call buttons is a constant issue in nursing homes. In fact, it is essentially ubiquitous. Not answering, or delaying in answering, the call button is so common, it is almost just an accepted feature of nursing home life. While there are times when calls might all be answered promptly, and there are certainly nurses who intend to answer calls promptly, the fact is it is unlikely any nursing home always answers every call quickly all the time.

Verbal Abuse and Humiliation

Our final category involves a common thread of dismissiveness, abuse, and humiliation that runs through much of what has been discussed above.

First of all, there is significant verbal abuse in the nursing home, coming from staff and directed at residents. Put simply, some staff are just plain mean, mean-spirited, vindictive, and cruel. The language and tone used to speak with those they are hired and paid to care for is repulsive. There can be quite a bit of yelling at residents, which we have sometimes caught on camera. This often goes hand-in-hand with the rough and aggressive behavior mentioned above. While some amount of frustration might be understandable in the job of nursing home staff, the use of yelling, threats, or other verbal abuse is simply inexcusable.

Another, even more malicious issue can be the use of direct humiliation regarding the residents. Taking photos of residents in humiliating fashion, mocking them, or laughing at them is all very common in this environment.

* * *

The issues raised in this and the last chapter cover a vast amount of territory in regards to what your loved one could experience. It is important to point out that not all residents suffer from any of these. At the same time, some residents may suffer from many of the above issues all at once.

That is why you must remain so vigilant over your loved one's care, not just in their general health but in the overall care and attention they are receiving. Some of these issues are more intentional and malicious than others, some are the fault of the nursing home and some not (more on that in the next section). Regardless, if you want your family member to live as healthy and happy a life as possible in the nursing home, you must remain aware of what can go wrong and watch out for it.

PART III

WHAT TO DO IF YOU SUSPECT SOMETHING IS WRONG

Chapter 6

Was This an Accident or Not?

AS ALWAYS, getting prompt medical attention is the number one priority for anyone after an injury. Legal aspects only come into play after you first receive medical care.

From a legal standpoint, some of the above categories of neglect and abuse are obvious cases in which the nursing home is guilty of negligence or even purposeful and malicious action against a resident. While all of those situations may not always lead to lawsuits, you can be confident that any verbal abuse or humiliation is definitely the nursing home's fault, and you should take immediate steps to protect your loved one and seek any justice you can.

However, not every category above is always so clear cut. Is a fall necessarily the nursing home's fault? Can't it just be an accident?

Before we answer that, let's back up a moment and reframe the question. It's better not to think of falls and other incidents as either accidents or not. Instead, we should think of them as either avoidable or unavoidable.

Every fall may be, in some sense, an accident (unless someone directly pushes another), but that does not mean it had to happen. When you are looking at the incidents that happen to your family member, try to keep that distinction in mind. Do not let the nursing home tell you the incident was an accident and it's no one's fault. Instead, think about whether the nursing home was doing enough to make sure such "accidents" do not happen in the first place.

Falls

We start with falls because it is often very difficult to know if they were due to nursing home neglect or just the byproduct of getting old. After all, many of the elderly have fragile bones and are unstable walkers. Some amount of falling, it seems almost intuitive, should be expected, right?

Actually, our intuition, in this case, is probably wrong. We have found that most falls in a nursing home were preventable. If the right protocols and tools had been put into place, most of those who have fallen and injured themselves would not have done so.

What we find in most of these cases is that the nursing home is not providing the best quality of care. Basically, what the nursing home is supposed to be doing, they are not doing. Often, this is because nursing homes are chronically short staffed, and so, they do not have the number of people to really watch everybody and make sure that the care plans they have implemented are actually being followed through with.

So, when you get a call that your loved one has fallen, how do you know whether it was avoidable or not?

The answer to that begins with your family member's admission assessment. As previously mentioned, when somebody enters the nursing home, they are assessed usually within the first 24 hours to see what specific needs are required to keep them safe. Part of every assessment is whether somebody is at risk of falling.

There are several factors that qualify somebody as a fall risk, some of which we discussed in the previous chapter. Essentially, those who need some assistance with their mobility (whether a walker or wheelchair) and those who are immobile are at the greatest risk. If that resident is at risk, then their care plan must take all reasonable steps to limit or reduce the risk of falling.

If this applies to your loved one, they should already be on a care plan that includes several ways to minimize this risk. As we discussed in the previous chapter, one of the common precautions taken against falling is lowering a bed toward the ground. That way, if there is a fall, the risk of injury is minimal. Another option is to have mats on the floor. Those who are at the highest risk can also be placed in rooms that are closer to the nursing stations, so that if they get up, the staff is close to provide assistance when the resident is unstable.

Residents should also have easy and comfortable access to their wheelchair, walker, or cane. It should always be placed closed by their bed, and assistance should be there any time it's needed. Often, residents require assistance in all transfers between a bed and a wheelchair. Therefore, the call button has to be within reach so they can call and get the required assistance to minimize the risk of falling.

Other care plan possibilities can only be implemented in certain situations. Bed rails on the bed, for instance, can run up against some difficulties in use because they are seen as a type of restraint in many states. In such situations, a doctor needs to sign off on them as a necessity. These same concerns are found in the use of lap belts while in a wheelchair.

Another care plan option is an alarm, although there is some controversy about whether it is effective or not. The controversy stems from the fact that an alarm does not actually prevent falls. Instead, they can minimize the risk of somebody falling by alerting nurses when they are out of bed. If somebody gets out of bed, and there's no alarm, they may get up and walk to the bathroom or exit the room without anyone knowing they are out of bed. This leaves a lot of time for potential falls. The alarm, then, gives the nursing home notification that somebody who shouldn't be out of bed unassisted has gotten out of bed. Therefore, someone can get to their room to hopefully prevent them from falling.

Obviously, it would be nearly impossible and cost prohibitive to watch any particular resident 24 hours a day, seven days a week, but that is never the goal of nursing home fall care plans. Instead, the goal with a fall-focused care plan is to minimize the risk and minimize the potential for injury.

So, when a fall occurs, the first step is to see whether the fall care plan was being followed completely. This usually requires the help of a lawyer, so it's best for you to contact one immediately after a fall takes place. Your lawyer can then advise you best on how to proceed.

This will involve checking every aspect of the care plan. Sometimes, lawyers discover that the resident was not properly assessed, and therefore, there was no care plan to prevent falls. Other times, we find that the care plan is not adequate for that specific resident. We have seen many instances in which somebody has had multiple falls and yet the care plan was not updated to reflect this new or heightened risk. After a fall, the nursing home must reassess the resident and update the care plan if needed. When adjustments are not made, this may prove that the nursing home did not do all it could to avoid the next fall.

Once the care plan is reviewed, steps are taken to see if the nursing home has been implementing the care plan fully in practice. For instance, one common fall risk involves nursing homes that have failed with their property upkeep. You can look for these sorts of issues with your own eyes. See if you can spot defects in the property that could be tripping hazards. You can also try to find out where the nurses place your family member's wheelchair or walking device to see if it is at an appropriate distance. Use your phone and take pictures.

It is important to note that falls are not always the fault of the nursing home. Sometimes, after all, an elderly person suffers a broken hip, and there is no real cause for it other than weakening bones. This weakening can lead to a fall that would be unavoidable.

There are also those residents who simply do not follow instructions. They are mentally competent, and the nursing home tells them not to get out of bed on their own. Yet, they choose to do it anyway. When they fall, it is more difficult to lay fault on the nursing home. If your loved one decides to get up because they think they have the strength—and they are competent to make that decision—and they then fall, it may not be the fault of the nursing home.

To get back to our main question: What should you do if the nursing home calls you and tells you that your family member had a fall? The simple answer is you need to go to the nursing home and see your loved one for yourself. You are the best person to recognize a change in their condition. If you feel the fall was serious, you should get experts involved.

You should also insist your loved one be taken to the hospital. Many times, we have had family members demand that their loved one be sent to the hospital, even when the nursing home claims they are fine. At the hospital, doctors then find out that they are, in fact, not fine and either have a broken bone or head injury.

Bedsores

Determining whether a bedsore is avoidable or unavoidable is very difficult and often requires the expertise of both a medical and legal review (as the standard used by a doctor and a lawyer may be different under the law). However, there are certainly many warning signs and factors that can point to a situation in which the bedsore was avoidable and the nursing home is to blame for allowing the development of this potentially painful and deadly skin issue.

The first determination is to confirm the skin issue your family member has is in fact a bedsore or pressure injury. Many wounds may look like a bedsore but are more properly classified as ischemic wounds. Ischemic, or vascular, wounds fool many of those who call our law firm, making them think an injustice has been done when that is not necessarily the case at all.

The reason ischemic wounds are confusing to people is because they look quite similar to bedsores. However, ischemic wounds are more often found not on pressure points (like the low back) but on the lower extremities, including the legs and feet. If the wound is on the front/top of the leg, it is more likely an ischemic wound and not a pressure wound. The major difference between the two, from a legal point of view, is how the wounds form. Bedsores come from unrelieved pressure on a part of the body that is supporting the body's weight, often caused by nursing home neglect. Ischemic wounds are due to poor blood circulation and not usually nursing home neglect.

Ischemic wounds often develop in those with diabetes or Peripheral Vascular Disease (PVD). Such wounds become very difficult to treat and to prevent, and they're generally not caused solely by nursing home neglect or abuse.

One area of the body in particular that is difficult to diagnose one way or the other is the heel. Generally speaking, when somebody who is diabetic or suffers from other vascular issues develops a heel wound, it is very difficult to pinpoint whether the wound was due to a nursing home's neglect in failing to remove the pressure or just the somewhat inevitable result of advanced circulatory problems.

In practice, both kinds of wounds on the heel can look the same. That is why it is rare for a nursing home law firm to take a case that only involves a wound on the heel. It is just too difficult to prove why it formed. While as a family member you may feel it best to move your loved one to ensure better care if such a wound develops, a lawsuit may be difficult to prove the cause.

However, when a wound is definitely a bedsore, it is, once again, often avoidable. Most bedsores that are formed at the nursing home on the buttock, sacral, or hips may have been avoidable. The first question is whether the resident was properly assessed as being a high risk for development of this wound. Does the resident have the physical strength or ability to turn and reposition themselves? If not, they may be at risk. Was a care plan initiated to prevent skin breakdown? Was a turning and reposition schedule in place or was the resident provided with a special mattress to help relieve pressure? In addition, and just as important, was a proper nutritional plan implemented to help prevent and promote healing of any skin issues?

Bedsores, and the prevention of them, are complex. At times, bedsores are unavoidable. Consider those who are hospitalized and on a breathing machine or other equipment that can't be turned off or removed. It becomes incredibly challenging to turn that individual every two hours because too much movement might endanger them in a different way. That would be a scenario in which a bedsore is almost unavoidable. It is hard to fault the staff in such an instance.

Another such situation is cancer treatment. Some cancer treatments can make skin become very fragile. This can lead to residents developing bedsores even with the best of care.

A final scenario that provides more complication is when a resident already has a bedsore or some other wound on a pressure point. From then onwards, there are only limited ways they can be moved. Say a resident has a wound on their lower back and are then moved between their left and right hip. This may increase the chance the left side develops a wound, and from there, the right side as well since there are fewer and fewer ways to reposition them. If the nursing home wasn't responsible for that initial wound, they may not be entirely responsible if another develops afterward. Again, this would depend upon a review to ensure that a proper turning and repositioning schedule was in place and implemented.

An extra lens through which to consider bedsores is not just whether they are avoidable or not, then, but also intention. If the nursing home did all it could with the intention of keeping a resident from developing bedsores, it can be difficult to assign them blame.

All that being said, it is still the case that the vast majority of bedsores that develop are avoidable, so if your loved one develops one, you ought to start by assuming that is the case until you can be convinced by a nursing home lawyer or a doctor otherwise.

Infections

Of the three categories introduced in Chapter 4, infections are perhaps the hardest to nail down as avoidable or unavoidable. The truth is, infections like pneumonia are very common in a nursing home setting. It does not require any especial neglect to allow it to spread.

That is the case at least if we consider the legal standard for neglect. However, if your family member is continually getting ill, that is a sign the nursing home isn't keeping the location as clean and sanitary as they should. They may also not be taking the precautions they should when an infection first presents itself.

However, that does not always mean the nursing home is not at fault for infections. We discussed in Chapter 4 how C-diff and UTIs can develop due to neglect on the part of the nursing home when they do not isolate those with the infection or remove catheters at an appropriate time.

Aspirational pneumonia can also be due to this same sort of carelessness. For those on a feeding tube, there is a greater risk of this infection when nurses don't raise the head of the bed enough during feedings or set the feeding tube at too fast a speed. If a nurse has the feeding tube on while a resident is lying flat, it can cause the tube to feed into the lungs, which can then cause aspiration pneumonia. That would require immediate hospitalization and can be fatal. In such a situation, the nursing home may be at fault.

A further concern with aspiration pneumonia is when residents choke and do not have the ability to cough out what they are choking on. If the nursing home does not provide assistance, that phlegm or food can end up in the lungs, which leads to the same result. This, though, may be harder to prove that the previous situation.

These examples just go to show that infection is complicated. As a general rule, it is best to accept that some amount of infection is likely for those who enter a nursing home, but always try to remain on top of any serious risks. Ask for updates on cases of pneumonia and C-diff in the nursing home. Ask to be informed if your loved one ever presents a fever, and if that fever doesn't go down in a few days, be prepared to demand more drastic action be taken.

Other categories

The other categories of neglect and abuse that are described in Chapter 5 are a bit easier to parse than falls, bedsores, and infections. Obviously, physical, sexual, and verbal abuse are all intentional and should be avoidable. Likewise, theft, overmedication, and the other topics covered. However, that does not mean they can be easily proven, especially at the level required in a legal case. We will cover that more in Part 4 of this book.

* * *

In general, when considering falls, bedsores, and infections, it is important to accept that few incidents are 100 percent clear when it comes to the avoidable/unavoidable line in a nursing home. Most of the time, they are preventable, but that is not always the case. It's best to think in these situations, "probably, but not necessarily."

However, you should treat any and every questionable incident the same way as those you are certain about. After medical attention has been provided, you should contact a nursing home lawyer immediately thereafter to protect the rights of your loved ones.

Chapter 7

How Do You Know If Your Family Member Is Being Abused or Neglected?

AS YOU CAN SEE from our previous discussion, it is not always clear when a nursing home is negligent. If you choose to contact a nursing home attorney with your questions, they can help sort out these difficult scenarios and provide you guidance. This is why there are nursing home attorneys for you to call.

Many times, abuse or neglect is happening in front of us and we do not even realize it, especially if there has not been any specific catastrophic event. Even in the case of a catastrophe, many nursing homes play down the severity of the situation because they fear your response.

So, how do you know if your family member has a bedsore? More importantly, how do you know before it's too late?

The answer to these questions is multifaceted and involves a number of different areas of vigilance. The first step is to know what risk factors affect your loved one so you can prioritize what to look for and worry about most. If you have a family member who is not able to turn and move around in bed by themselves, they are going to be at risk of a bedsore. Therefore, take all available steps to limit that risk.

Start by talking to the nursing home staff to learn as much as possible about the care plan put into place for your loved one and attend all care plan meetings. Call regularly to make sure that the nurses, aides, and doctors are checking your loved one for any signs of skin breakdown. Then, when visiting, physically check and look yourself for any skin issues. As is always the case, you want to visit your family member as often as possible, and every time you visit conduct an examination.

Every visit may seem extreme to some, but it is very important to be so focused on this. The nursing home is supposed to call you when there is a change in condition, including any type of skin breakdown. You are supposed to get notified. However, do not rely on the receiving of this call; it may not come. Therefore, every time you visit, do a thorough body check to make sure nothing has gone unreported. Even though it may be uncomfortable looking at your mother's or father's body parts, it is something that needs to be done because it could be fatal otherwise.

Even if the nursing home calls you and properly reports that your family member has developed a bedsore, you still need to go and look at it yourself. Do not just expect the nursing home to be forthright. We have found, time and time again, that the nursing home will downplay very serious bedsores and make them sound like it's no big deal. "It's small." "It's minor." "It's being treated." "It's already healing." "Nothing to worry about." These sorts of expressions lure many family members into a complacency that can be catastrophic and painful for a resident. By the time a visit is made and the bedsore examined, a huge and infected wound is discovered, not the small, healing, nothing to worry about skin issue that was reported.

Far too often, we are told by family members of recently deceased or critically ill residents that they were told everything was going to be alright repeatedly. Because of such confidence and certainty, our clients simply forget about the issue for a time. They stop asking questions because they were told the wound is healing and improving. Then, tragically, a few months later, our clients learn that their loved one is in the hospital, and the doctors ask them, "Did you know that your mom has this gigantic, Stage 4, infected bedsore?"

Our best advice to anyone who is told by the nursing home staff that a bedsore has developed is to immediately visit, examine, and take a photo of the wound. You need to see and document it on your own. If you regularly visit your family member, you will have a good level of appreciation for the change in their condition.

Another benefit of regular checks is the ability to find out what the nursing home may be hiding. Sometimes, nursing homes go beyond not reporting the beginnings of a bedsore; they actually hide it. You may visit and find bandages at a pressure point on your loved one's body without any explanation or notification. If you see bandages anywhere on your loved one, insist on an explanation. You may not be able to see the wounds due to the bandages but you can ask the nurse to tell you the stage and size of the wound. Then, continue to ask about it on a regular, weekly basis. If possible, that is also a good time to increase the frequency of your visits.

If there is a bedsore, the nursing home is supposed to measure the wound every week, and wound care professionals should be treating it. Therefore, you should be getting updates on a regular basis describing how the bedsore is progressing and whether the size is getting larger or smaller. Again, do not just trust the updates. After those nurse notifications, you want to keep an eye on it yourself as much as possible.

A final and very important point on bedsores: once your loved one develops a bedsore, you should call a lawyer. As you already know by now, many times, bedsores are due to neglect, and you need a lawyer's advice to know how to move forward and what legal options are best for your family member.

You may also, either before or after speaking to a lawyer, try to get an outside doctor's opinion. While the nursing home should either have doctors on staff or have doctors that regularly visit. Getting another opinion just further clarifies the nature of your loved one's situation and your options. That information can help your lawyer as well.

Much of the bedsore advice above also applies for other major health issues in the nursing home. If your loved one is a fall risk, make sure all the proper precautions are in place and visit as much as possible to make sure the care plan is being followed. If a fall does take place, do not just take the nursing home's word that your family was not injured. Speak to your family member and visit immediately.

Too many times to count, family members were told their loved one was not injured after a fall and is doing just fine. Sadly, when the family visits, they find their loved one with severe black and blue faces and horrible bruises.

Often, these bruises turn out to be more than just bruises. There may be broken bones involved that the nursing home failed to assess because they did not send the resident to the hospital. In that situation, the family really must step in to insist on proper and immediate medical care and attention.

Falls and bedsores usually show signs of occurrence. Other injuries or issues of neglect or abuse are sometimes harder to pinpoint and require more focused attention.

In particular, watch out for sudden changes in behavior, loss of weight, or a sudden decline in health. These are common signs that something is not being done correctly. Since many nursing home residents are incapable of directly saying something is wrong—due to Alzheimer's, dementia, or other conditions—families must look for these secondary signs.

Often, abuse only manifests through such indirect signs.

One new and incredibly useful way to get a much better appreciation for how your loved one is being treated: cameras. The ability to use a video camera depends on state laws.

To take the example of one state, Illinois has recently allowed family members of residents to put cameras in their loved one's room to monitor them. Among the requirements, though, is the need to post a notification outside of the room to warn people that they are entering a space that is recorded. The state also requires any roommates to sign off on the use of a camera to protect their own privacy.

If you can get through the loopholes, video cameras are a great way to protect against wrong-doing, discover if wrong-doing is occurring, and collect evidence of wrong-doing if the need for legal action arises. As this technology becomes more prevalent, more states are likely to make it legal, so be sure to find out if it is allowed where you live.

The other and best way to find out if something is going wrong is to be there yourself. Personally checking on a resident's care is ideal. However, with busy schedules, it can be difficult. We recommend, if possible, to have different family members come and visit at different times of the day. Try to avoid getting into a regular schedule as the nursing home staff will pick up on it if you always visit your mom after work on Tuesdays and Thursdays. So, on Tuesdays and Thursdays, your mom may look like she's getting great care. She looks her best: clean and healthy. But you don't know what's going on the rest of the time.

If you have other family members who can make these trips at different hours, ask them to do so with some regularity as well. This forces nursing homes to always be prepared for a visit, even from someone they don't recognize. It means they can't afford to let your loved one's care slip.

In summation, then, the best ways to find out if your loved one in a nursing home is being neglected or abused are:

- Do not wait for the nursing home to tell you. They may not, or they may only tell you part of it. Go and find out everything for yourself.
- Insist on seeing a doctor or going to the hospital when something happens, even if the nursing home says it is not necessary.
- Watch for changes in body, activity, emotional state, etc.
- Use whatever methods are legal to supervise your loved one as much as possible.
- Mix up your schedule and visit at different times of the day and week to see how your loved one is being treated. Also, have other family members visit using the same system.
- Always be ready to call a lawyer. Save the lawyer's number in your phone in case a call is needed.

Chapter 8

Changing Nursing Homes—

How, When, and Why?

OUR LAW FIRM gets a lot of questions about how, when, and why to move or change nursing homes. These are difficult questions to answer because there are personal, as well as medical, legal, and practical implications.

At the same time, this question, when it arises in our context, is actually two questions: If I want to change nursing homes, how do I go about it? And, do I have to change nursing homes if I'm going to bring a lawsuit?

To address the first question first: it is worth pointing out that you have every right to move nursing homes at any time. There are no laws requiring you stay in one facility, and Medicaid will allow residents to change without it affecting coverage. The trick, then, is not the right to move but finding a better place. It can be a real challenge to find a better home, especially one with an immediately available bed that can take your family member. Finding a new home, after all, is at least as difficult as finding that first home (which we discussed in Chapter 3). The new home still has to be able to meet all of the medical needs of your loved one. It still needs to be close enough to you that you can visit relatively easily. It still needs to pass all the tests you set for it, especially the gut feeling test.

If you do find a new home (or a few potential options) you are comfortable with, you still need to figure out the logistics. In other words, you need to figure out the "how" in changing homes. For this, we recommend trying to switch nursing homes during a hospitalization. This is usually the easiest way to make the change. At that point, the hospital social worker and staff can provide assistance in finding an available home. These same individuals should also be able to ensure your loved one's future nursing home can handle their specific care needs. This is important because even though the care is bad at the current home, you do not want to just up and move your family member to a place that is not capable of handling their very serious medical needs. If they need dialysis or tracheotomy care, make sure the new location has the ability to handle those needs. Once more, to learn more about this, we recommend you reread Chapter 3.

Another reason we recommend switching nursing homes while your loved one is at the hospital is the logistic ease, as they are already physically out of the home. So, it is an easy transfer for them because they are going from the hospital directly to the new home.

However, be prepared, as often there are delays or barriers when getting into the desired home. The system does not always work perfectly. Some potential barriers may depend upon your family member's billing scenario. Do you need a Medicare or Medicaid bed or a specific insurance bed? For example, the nursing home you wish to transfer to may have limited number of Medicaid beds and, therefore, may not be available at the time you need. If no beds are available, you can always get on a waiting list and wait it out at the home your loved one is currently in until a bed becomes available, but that can be a long wait.

We already know that finding a home with a free bed, with the right specializations for your family member, and at the right location is key to keeping your family member safe and healthy. Unfortunately, checking all of those boxes is not always easy. Depending on where you live, how close you need your loved one to be, their special needs, and their financial situation, the wait could be nonexistent, or it could be years.

A significant factor in finding an available home often comes down to a matter of geography. In some communities, particularly in and around big cities, it is fairly easy to find another available home that fits your family member's needs. For those in smaller, more remote communities with few nursing home options, though, it can take a great deal of time. We have had clients who waited over a year before a bed opened up, but most clients are able to move their loved ones to a new home without any interruption.

As mentioned above, in an ideal situation, you will find a new nursing home while in the hospital and transfer your loved one straight from the hospital to the new nursing facility. In this scenario, your family member never has to return to the place where they were harmed. However, it is just as possible, and just as common, to transfer from one nursing home straight to another nursing home. A transfer from nursing home to nursing home has the benefit of time. You can take as long as needed.

In the end, the choice is a matter of financial options, comfort, availability, and simply what is possible.

Now, to move on to our second question of this chapter: Should you move your family member in the case of a lawsuit? The answer is yes, usually. To begin with, if you are concerned enough about the quality of care your loved one is receiving that you have hired a nursing home lawyer, you should move your family member to a new facility for their safety and well-being.

That is just based on concern for their safety and comfort. A lawsuit suggests something serious has happened, that your loved one was severally injured, neglected, or abused. Finding a new home is probably the best choice.

There is also a second reason to move your loved one: it simply looks bad for your case if they stay. If your case ever gets in front of a jury, the jury may look at your loved one and wonder if the situation can be as bad as we describe it since you have stuck with the same nursing home. According to this thinking, if you are so unhappy with the care, and you feel that your loved one is in such danger, you would have done anything to change the situation. Of course, we can (and do) argue extenuating circumstances, but it's easier for your case if a move is made.

So, for both of those reasons, we recommend that you move your family member. That being said, there have been many situations where a move is not possible or not in the best interest of the loved one. As previously discussed, in some situations there are no available homes that meet your family's needs. In other cases, the need to move is not urgent, as the incident that led to a lawsuit was isolated, or important factors have changed, like the negligent staff is no longer working at the facility. We have also seen a few instances where the staff at the same nursing home tries to pay extra attention, knowing that your loved one has suffered harm at their doing. The staff tries to actively provide better care.

Others choose not to move because their family member is, overall, quite comfortable in that home, and a move might be too traumatic for them. This is often the case for those who suffer with Alzheimer's or dementia. In their fragile state, moving would likely cause a dramatic impact on their overall well-being and comfort.

A final consideration is location. When the current facility is very close to you and all alternatives facilities are significantly farther, it can end up being a very tough decision, and remaining close may be the better choice. The ability to visit more often at the close location can ensure better treatment than to risk a move where you are unable to visit regularly.

For those who decide moving is not right for them, we recommend reaching out to your local ombudsman. Long-term ombudsmen are advocates for residents in nursing homes and assisted living communities that handle complaints. It is a free service provided by the government. An ombudsman is available to settle smaller disputes that do not reach the level of a lawsuit. The ombudsman is essentially the middle person between the nursing home and the residents.

However, while this is a great resource, remember that an ombudsman does not work for you. Unlike a lawyer that is always on your side, the ombudsman is supposed to be a neutral party that focuses on how to resolve any issues between the two sides.

This can be a very useful tool when a situation does not concern the safety of your loved one or rise to the level of a lawsuit. For concerns over changing rooms, shower schedules, missing clothes or items, or other complaints about part of their care that doesn't rise to the level of abuse or neglect, the ombudsman is there to help reach a compromise.

Perhaps the best way to think of the ombudsman is as the step to take when your loved one does not want to move or when treatment has not resulted in harm.

However, whether you think you want to work with the nursing home to find a solution or you want to get out as soon as possible, if events have taken place that have made life difficult for your loved one, it's always best to contact a nursing home lawyer for answers to your questions. A nursing home lawyer will be able to help you work through your options. They can let you know whether the nursing home's actions rise to the level of abuse or neglect.

Better decisions are made with better information. So utilize a free phone call to a nursing home lawyer to help with your concerns or questions about whether you should transfer homes.

PART IV

HOW TO PURSUE LEGAL ACTION

Chapter 9

How Much Will It Cost?

And Other Questions Answered

IF YOU HAVE REACHED THIS POINT in the book, you are probably already facing a very difficult nursing home situation. Your loved one has been harmed in some way, either abused or neglected. Understandably, you have a lot of questions about what to do. In particular, you want to know if you should get a lawyer and what that process will look like. This fourth and final section is designed to answer all of your questions so you know what to expect today, tomorrow, and a year down the line.

In this first chapter of Part 4, we lay out some of the most common questions we hear from those who call us about incidents in the nursing home.

How much does it cost to hire an attorney?

All attorneys' fees are contingent upon a settlement. What that means is the family will never have to pay anything out of pocket at any time, ever, to hire a lawyer. If a settlement is reached, attorney's fees are set by contract with limitations imposed in many states. They usually range between 33.3 and 40 percent of the settlement.

If we lose the case, do we have to pay?

In almost all states, you never pay anything unless you receive a settlement. There are a few states that may have special rules concerning fees. You may discuss the laws of your particular state with the lawyer.

As a general rule, there is zero financial risk for a family to hire an attorney and pursue a lawsuit in a nursing home case.

Is my loved one too old for a lawsuit?

Many people think there is a practical barrier against a lawsuit if their family member is over a certain age. The short answer to this is, no, there is no such barrier. However, some lawyers may still refuse the case for that reason. You will find that some attorneys are under the impression that juries will not sympathize with those who have lived past the age of life expectancy.

We do not share that opinion. We frequently represent clients of advanced ages. For example, we represented an 89-year-old man named Daniel Foresyte who developed a serious bedsore while getting rehab following hip surgery. That bedsore became infected and, unfortunately, led directly to his death four months later. We carried on the case in his honor and prevailed with a substantial settlement for his family.

We had another client, Sylvia Stein, who was a 90-year-old resident with dementia when she fell and broke her hip because the nursing home failed to fulfill its care plan. That case, even though she was 90, settled for $700,000.

Despite the advanced age of Daniel and Sylvia, we were still able to win them and their families very high settlement amounts. Their age had no bearing on our case values.

Our success in representing these clients of advanced age is based upon how we view these cases. Many lawyers will look at a case like Daniel's or Sylvia's and see an unsympathetic client. They often feel that, because of their advanced age, that death's door is nearby anyway. That thinking leads such lawyers to assume that a jury would not understand that the injured or deceased individual is still a loving being who has suffered. These lawyers think the decline or death of the very old is not as emotional as it would be if they were younger.

Our approach is that no one, no matter their age, should live their final days, months, or years with unnecessary pain and suffering. If they had to go through the last six months of their lives, even at age 89, dealing with an injury or a series of traumatic events all because of neglect or abuse, that upsets people. That perspective allows juries to see our clients as who they are: people who deserved better, and people with families who deserve justice. We also realize that holding a nursing home responsible financially will help those old residents receive the same quality care as younger residents.

Who can hire an attorney for a loved one?

We get a lot of phone calls from people who wish to pursue legal action on behalf of someone close to them. Unfortunately, closeness alone is not the determining factor for who can bring a case. So, who, exactly, can bring a case? This is somewhat complicated in nursing home law. For those residents who are alive and mentally competent, the resident themselves is the only person who can bring the case. If the nursing home resident is not competent—because, for instance, they have suffered a catastrophic stroke or suffer with dementia or Alzheimer's—the person who brings the suit must have power of attorney.

If there is no power of attorney, somebody must first be appointed as guardian to bring a lawsuit.

Ideally, the group of family members who contact an attorney will include the person with power of attorney or guardianship. The more the family is together on a case, the better, although we are able to work with those families that are not so ideally situated.

I want to bring a case, but my brother doesn't want to. Can I still bring a case?

Again, this question comes into play depending on who has power of attorney. As we mentioned above, ideally, we want all family members on board and working together. However, if there is disagreement, so long as you have power of attorney, you can go ahead with the case. You do not need the entire family's permission to bring a case.

If my sister hires attorney, do I need to get my own lawyer?

No, you should only have one lawyer handling the case. Only one person should be in control of the lawsuit, so there should only be one law firm handling the case.

Does my family member have to leave the nursing home if we pursue a case?

As we discussed in Chapter 8, it is generally recommended that the family move a resident if they are going to pursue a case, but it's certainly not required. The thought process on the legal side is that a jury will be less sympathetic to your situation if you did not feel what happened was serious enough to require changing homes.

If your loved one is still at the target nursing home, it gives the impression that you are not so concerned about the wellbeing and safety of your loved one.

As previously mentioned in Chapter 8, there are many times when it is more harmful to move the resident to a new home. While deciding one way or the other, this usually has no immediate bearing on our ability to bring a lawsuit against the nursing home.

Some lawyers will choose not to bring a case if the family will not move a loved one, but we feel that the lawyer should not try to force that issue. We respect the family's decisions and will work with whatever you feel is best for your family member, so long as they have maximum comfort and safety.

A final wrinkle is that, on rare occasions, settlements require a resident to move. Nursing homes do, at times, ask that a resident be moved to a different facility. It is not very common, but it does occur. Usually, though, the settlement is more than large enough to cover this inconvenience.

Can the nursing home kick my loved one out for filing a suit?

No. Beyond asking for it in a settlement, they cannot legally kick your family member out. However, some nursing homes may try to find other reasons to have your loved one leave. For example, they may send them to a hospital claiming the resident is a risk of harm to the other residents.

What if the nursing home changes their records? How do we prove that? Does that hurt our case?

There's always a risk the nursing home might try to change records, and we look closely to see if we can find any such changes. It does happen, but not often. Also, as technology advances in record keeping, falsifying records are becoming much more difficult for nursing homes.

We are able to catch changes through our access to multiple copies of records. We compare records we receive at different times and records from different sources to see if changes have been made.

When we do discover record changes, this does not harm our client's case at all. Quite the opposite, in fact. It is actually very harmful to the nursing home. A confirmed falsified record usually helps our client's cases and negatively affects the home's case. It can highlight the nursing home's guilt. In our experience, it also really raises a jury's anger at the nursing home, which leads to larger results.

However, changing records does not happen as often as families think it does.

How much is my case worth?

This is, of course, a very common question. Unfortunately, it is also a very difficult one for us to answer, especially at the beginning of the case. The truth is, before we have all the facts, it is simply impossible to know how much a case is worth. Until we have thoroughly reviewed the case and understand the other side's position, it serves no purpose to speculate on a value. It is a very bad practice.

Speculating on a case's value without all available information causes harm to the attorney-client relationship without adding any benefit. If the estimated case value seems too low, some clients will be hesitant to move forward, even if the final settlement ends up being much higher. If, on the other hand, the initial value is too high and additional facts learned later lower the ultimate value of the case, the client will never forget that first number. The client may then feel disappointed with the settlement or resolution. They may feel that the attorney has failed them, despite a successful settlement. Whether too high or too low, that first number tends to stick in people's minds, and it makes it difficult to approach the case properly when a number is already floating around.

The truth is, there is no way any attorney can know on day one what a case is worth. A lot of factors come into play over the course of a case that can make a potential value fluctuate. The proper time to discuss case value is after the case has been fully reviewed and assessed.

Even giving a ballpark is difficult with nursing home cases. While most settlements fall somewhere in the six figures, some are much higher and others somewhat lower.

While we understand this can be frustrating, we act this way for the benefit of all sides. In fact, it should raise immediate concerns if a lawyer offers you a high settlement figure upfront without thoroughly reviewing your case. Some attorneys will use this tactic to lure in clients, only to change the value later. They give prospective clients the big number they want to hear so the client will hire them. Then, as the case progresses, the client will learn that the true value is not what was originally sold to them. It is our opinion that this is not a proper or ethical way for an attorney to represent their clients.

Who receives the settlement money?

If the resident is alive, the money goes to them (if they are mentally competent) or to the power of attorney (if they are not). In that case, it is still, technically, the resident's money. The person with power of attorney just manages it for the resident. The person with power of attorney is not allowed to use the money for their own personal purposes.

After a resident's death, the money is disbursed to the resident's estate.

Can I be blamed since I placed my family in a nursing home?

No. Nursing homes provide an important service in our country. When someone needs around-the-clock care with complex medical needs, keeping them at home without trained staff is not feasible. Nursing homes are needed. While, sometimes, the nursing home defendant will try to cast blame on the family, we find this is not an effective or honest tactic. Many of our clients come to us feeling guilty and responsible for what happened to their relative in the nursing home, but it is neither legally nor morally their fault. It was the actions of others that harmed their loved one, not their choice to entrust them to expert care.

You were told, when you placed your family member in a nursing home, something like, "This is what we do. We can take good care of your mom." Or, "Now your father will get the care he needs." Then, they failed you. The guilt is all on them.

What if the resident dies before the case is resolved? What happens to the case?

If the resident dies during the duration of the case, the case continues. A family member will be appointed as the administrator or executor of the estate and the case proceeds on behalf of the estate of the resident.

How long does the case take?

A nursing home case generally takes several years to resolve. Depending on the jurisdiction and the state, the duration of a case varies. On average and depending on your state, most cases take between two to four years to resolve.

What if the state complaint came back with no violations, can we still pursue a case?

Yes. A case can and should be pursued despite a no violation finding from the state. We recommend that all of our clients file a complaint against the nursing home with their state's Department of Health, or whichever agency oversees nursing homes. Despite the amount of negligence and abuse that occurs in these homes, we find that most of our cases shockingly receive a no violation letter from the state's investigation. The truth is, if we only took cases that came back with violations, it would falsely appear that thousands of neglected or abused residents received proper care when they did not.

If the state's surveyor found no neglect or improper nursing care in your case, this does not mean that there's no grounds for a lawsuit. The state's investigation varies in quality, and it is greatly dependent upon the specific surveyor. We find that some surveyors perform a very thorough investigation and are more likely find issues of neglect or improper case. Meanwhile, we find other surveyors just seem to walk in, take a glance around, assume everything's fine, and turn around and leave. The findings are just one very minor factor used in assessing your case, and they are not heavily relayed upon.

So, why do we still strongly recommend that you notify the state of your complaint? In addition to a finding of neglect helping your case, we recommend the filing of a complaint as a public service. Whenever a complaint is filed with the state, it is posted to the state's website without the names. This is a great resource for other families to look up and see how many complaints have been filed against this home. This may help make sure the next family looking for a nursing home does not become the next victim.

If we win the case, will my mother lose her Medicaid benefits? Do we have to pay back Medicaid?

As Medicaid is a state benefit, the laws surrounding Medicaid rights and reimbursement are state specific, and you will need to discuss these issues and concerns directly with a nursing home attorney. In general, if you obtain a settlement or verdict on behalf of a Medicaid beneficiary, depending on the amount of the settlement, it could impact your loved one's benefits. There are certain procedures and trusts that can be established to ensure those benefits are not impacted, but again, this is a state specific law.

If the nursing home is no longer in business, can we still file a case?

Generally speaking, we can, but it depends on whether the nursing home is covered by insurance. It is best to consult an attorney on the specific nursing home to see if a lawsuit is feasible.

If I already have an attorney but I'm not happy with them, can I switch and will that cost me money?

Yes, if you already have an attorney on the case and you're not happy, another lawyer can take it over. There is no cost to the client to switch attorneys.

It is pretty common for a client to switch attorneys, whether because of false promises like those mentioned earlier in this chapter, a lack of communication (such as a failure to return phone calls), or just a sense the lawyer is not making the proper effort on a particular case.

No matter your reasoning, switching attorneys is very easy for the client. Your new lawyer should handle the entire process for you. You, as the client, only need to sign a letter of direction. There are no additional costs or fees that are incurred. Depending on the amount of work the first lawyer performed on the case, they may be entitled to share in part of the attorney's fees, but the total fee charged to you remains the same from your perspective.

Basically, that's a problem for lawyers to work out, not you. You always pay the same attorneys' fees on your case, whether you see the case through with one lawyer or not.

Chapter 10

Why Consider a Lawsuit?

ONE OF THE ISSUES we come across with our clients is a reluctance to begin the legal process. Hiring an attorney may feel like a major burden to the family. At the same time, many families feel guilty about placing their loved one in a home to begin with and assume they bear certain amount of responsibility. They feel foolish for having trusted the nursing home in the first place. And, besides, what good is going to come out of this?

The answer to that final question is: plenty of good, for many different people.

There are, in fact, many excellent reasons to file a lawsuit. In this chapter, we are going to highlight only a few of them. They may not be your reasons, but they are strong ones.

Let's start with the most fundamental aspect of a nursing home lawsuit: justice. If the nursing home has wronged you and your family, you have the right to bring a lawsuit and seek closure and compensation. This is a fundamental part of how our country and our system of justice operates. We do not let those who are guilty of harm continue with their bad behavior.

This point, though, is only the beginning of why you should pursue a lawsuit. Another significant argument is that lawsuits help produce change. Many of our clients express a desire to make sure what happened to their family never happens again. That admirable goal is perhaps impossible in a grand sense, but it does occur in a more limited way. There is only so much you can do to make a change when it comes to nursing homes. You can talk to legislators about changing the law, but that's a long, drawn out battle as well, and you may have only a limited effect without more powerful backers.

A more direct way to push for change is through the court, the judicial part of our society. Any type of verdict, even a settlement, is a negative from the nursing home's point of view. Going to court and having to pay money is obviously something they want to avoid. Since most nursing homes are for-profit, this can really hit them where it hurts them most: the bottom line. That can lead them to take immediate steps to avoid future lawsuits, which result in better care. A successful lawsuit sends a powerful message that this type of harm has got to stop in their institution. In that sense, the larger the settlement, the more they may feel compelled to make those changes.

These lawsuits also act as a warning for those families considering entering that nursing home. Families can search court records to learn how many lawsuits have been filed against a specific nursing home when searching for a home for their loved one. Hopefully, all families will do this, and if they see many complaints and lawsuits against a facility, they may think twice before entrusting their loved one to that same kind of care. Again, if the verdict is very high in your case, it might also get some media attention that would further spread the word about what the nursing home has done. This publicity may, in the end, help influence legislators to act and protect our elderly residents residing in these homes.

Even if not, the very threat of this possibility can be enough to promote change within the nursing home and the staffing issues.

In some cases, the desire to produce change can lead to some amazing and life-affirming changes. In Chapter 4, we introduced you to a woman named Martina, who developed bedsores at her nursing home and eventually died as a result.

Martina's daughter, Sophie, was the one who pursued the case on her behalf. Instead of just walking away with a substantial settlement, Sophie decided she needed to do something positive. She became so involved in what was happening with her mom, and so upset at what had occurred, that she ended up using the settlement money from the case to start a business dedicated to eradicating the problem.

Sophie's business—which continues to thrive many years after her case—hires people to go and visit the residents in nursing homes when the family is unable to visit as often as they would like. For those who are not able to visit on their own because of their work schedule or logistics, they can send somebody once a week, twice a week, or more. Whatever schedule they need, they can hire someone to go and just spend time with their family member. This is not a sitter system, which was already in place, it is something profoundly healthier. It's much more interactive and positive for the resident. These individuals are just friendly visitors who spend time with the resident, interacting with the resident, bringing them more joy and companionship. At the same time, they are undeniably useful as a separate pair of eyes to watch for signs of neglect or abuse, allowing others to avoid the horrors that Sophie and Martina experienced.

The positive benefits of Sophie's business from the emotional impact on the residents to the improved care with someone there to watch would not have been possible if Sophie had not pursued a lawsuit on her mother's behalf. She has undoubtedly improved hundreds of lives at this point, all because she had the courage to take a stand for Martina.

Many readers will surely find Sophie admirable but still feel very pessimistic about anyone's ability to change nursing home culture. That is understandable for those who are still dealing with the trauma of what has happened to them and to their loved ones, but it is worth pointing out that sometimes nursing homes do change, genuinely.

Sometimes, this change is by compulsion, either due to financial fears through lawsuits or due to the lawsuits themselves. We have seen firsthand how some nursing homes become convinced over time that they simply must have more staff, even when it cuts into their profits. That's a concrete change that happened because families stood up for those who were being harmed

Sometimes, though, a nursing home does change because it has seen the error of its ways. One of our recent cases involved a nursing home that actually offered to put a plaque up with the resident's name as a memorial and as a reminder of how they let her down.

It is important to note that while we may find that those running some nursing homes may not necessarily care about the residents, there are plenty of individuals working in those nursing homes who do care. We have seen nurses and Certified Nursing Assistants reach out personally to families with concern about the care received. These individuals have made attempts to improve the care and practices of their institution. That plaque was a great start, and we hope it leads to further change.

Nursing homes can learn their lesson, and nursing homes can improve, but that will only happen if they are confronted with the costs and expenses of lawsuits.

Another significant reason to pursue justice is closure. Closure is somewhat connected to the above two points. Many seek closure by pursuing justice for their family. Others seek closure by finding some way to achieve something positive, some form of change, out of a horrible event. Others, though, need to be able to see the full truth before they can move on, and we can often provide that.

Many times, a family comes to us not knowing what happened. They have a vague or contracted story and just know that something has gone wrong; they do not have any accurate details. This leads to a lot of stress and anxiety. Families often fill in the blanks with the worst possible events, or else, find ways to blame themselves.

We find that when family members understand and learn exactly what happened and get all the facts, they are able to achieve some sense of closure for themselves. It is a powerful thing to confront the truth, even when it is awful, but individuals in these situations do not have the power or knowledge to get to that truth on their own. They need us to find it for them.

The unknown can cause lot of anxiety; it can make it impossible to move on. Pursuing a case is something that you do on behalf of a family member who you love and who suffered. They may no longer have the ability to bring forth the case, to fight for themselves, but you are doing it for them.

The inability to protect those we love is a horrible feeling, however it is still possible to do something for them. When your loved one suffered due to the neglect or harm caused by someone, that someone should not get away with it. They should be held responsible for their actions and forced to confront those actions publicly.

Although these events may have happened to your mother or father and not directly to you, it is important to recognize that this is also a traumatic experience for you and for the rest of your family. You need to find the means to come to some amount of closure for your own benefit. You need to be able to move on at some point.

A final reason to pursue a case is financial. While your case is not about the money, money is one of the best ways we have in our system to improve the care of your loved one or motivate bad actors to operate as they promised at the time you trusted your loved one with them. You are entitled to money damages under the law. Their carelessness or negligence caused pain and suffering to your loved one and your family. Again, these lawsuits are the strongest motivation for nursing homes to improve the quality of care. We must not stop that fight.

The money received from these cases can now be used in many positive ways to better your family member's life, and to better your life. Settlements can be used to get a bed at another nursing home, for instance. The money might, under some circumstances, also be used to take a family member out of the nursing home and provide care at home. Some families use the money to move closer to their loved one in the nursing home, so that they are able to visit as often as possible, watching over their care and improving their day-to-day life. It might also be used to provide everyone with a well-deserved long vacation after such a difficult period.

That is only the beginning of what a settlement can do for you and your family. You can also use this settlement fund to donate to your favorite charity and help promote change in a more global sense. You may hold this money for the day another family member may need medical or nursing home care. There are many excellent organizations dedicated to helping stop the exact types of abuses your family member suffered.

Again, you and your family did your part in trusting the care of your loved one with a nursing home. Unfortunately, the nursing home failed your trust. You are the ones who have been hurt, and you have a legal right to compensation.

Chapter 11

How and When Should I Hire a Lawyer?

AT THIS POINT, it should be clear why contacting an attorney sooner rather than later is important.

Like almost all legal rights, you have a limited time to file a claim. In some states, it can be as short as one year. This time period is different in each state, may differ depending on case types, and may also depend upon your unique situation. No matter what the length may be, time is of the essence. Since these cases are often complicated and usually require a lot of medical record review before a lawsuit is filed, it is important that your contact an attorney promptly so that there is sufficient time to allow this review.

Investigating promptly is also important. Getting witness statements and taking the deposition of employees now instead of years from now may save your claim. People forget what they know or convey the wrong information due to lapses in memory. Your family member's roommate at the nursing home may provide critical information to support your case, but if you delay too long, that roommate may no longer be at that nursing home.

There is no harm to contact an attorney immediately after any injury. Nursing home lawyers do not charge for phone calls. You want to make the call so you can make informed decisions rather than guess. Better to be safe than sorry. Remember, as we learned in the last chapter, it does not cost anything to consult a lawyer. It does not cost anything to pursue a lawsuit. There's no good reason to delay, and a lot of reasons not to delay.

Also, delays may result in a change of the nursing staff. The staff at fault may be no longer be at the nursing home, and they may be difficult to track down.

How do you choose the right attorney? Begin by narrowing down your options. Look specifically for lawyers who focus their practice on handling nursing home cases. Nursing home cases are not like any other injury case. They are very different and very specialized. We have first-hand experience with this situation, as we have had many clients who have come to us after they were unsatisfied with their first choice of law firm.

What many of these attorneys who are unfamiliar with nursing home cases do not always understand or focus on is that in almost every nursing home case, we start with someone who is already in poor health, and that's why they are at the nursing home. Prior health issues are not an excuse for the nursing home to cause them more suffering. Just because they were already unwell doesn't mean it is okay to mistreat them.

That presentation must focus on how the nursing home failed. These cases are not only about what happened to your loved one, but why it happened. The why it happened is usually due to the nursing home's under-staffing and under-training. When nursing homes understaff the facilities, there simply are not enough care-takers to properly care for the resident's needs, and bad and deadly things will happen.

Nursing home owners and administrators know how many people are needed to properly care for the residents. They have the resources to provide the highest level of care to their residents. This information is publicly available. Medicare releases figures that relate how much staff nursing homes have versus how much money they are taking in. The ability is there, but nursing homes choose to cut corners when and where they shouldn't. It is this, frankly—cutting corners and neglecting care—that should be the focus of any nursing home lawsuit.

Most of the issues discussed in previous chapters that detail all the kinds of harm residents can sustain all come back to this under-staffing. Under-staffing leads to more residents falling because they do not receive support from staff. It leads to bedsores because there is not enough staff to timely turn all the residents. It leads to residents becoming dehydrated and malnourished because staff is not available to help them eat and drink. It leads to infections spreading because staff are unable to properly isolate and treat infections.

These issues can all occur despite a lack of malice on behalf of the staff; they are due to the nursing home simply refusing to hire the staff necessary to run the home.

During your first call to a law firm, listen and pay attention to how focused on your questions the attorney or person you first speak to is. Are they rushing you off the phone, or are they taking the time to hear your entire story and ask questions? Are they sympathetic? Do they care? Are all of your questions answered? Do they really listen to your story? If you are not talking with an attorney, do they offer you to speak with an attorney?

If an attorney will not give you the proper amount of time on the phone to answer all of your questions until you hire them, you need to find someone else. Trust is a crucial element of the attorney-client relationship.

You want to finish that first phone call feeling like the person you talked to understood you and your case, sympathized with you, and had the experience and knowledge to win your case. In other words, you want to finish that phone call trusting your new lawyer completely. You should have a feeling of relief, not like more stress was placed upon the situation.

We have seen some small firms or new firms that are unproven in the field that simply cannot afford to handle a nursing home case, no matter their intentions. There are a lot of expenses that the attorney must advance on the case in order to properly prepare your case. Lawyers must hire top-notch experts to review the information of your case. They also have to work for years without receiving any compensation. Some new or inexperienced small firms have yet to establish themselves enough to afford such major expenses. It's possible the money will simply run out to handle your case properly, which leads to corner-cutting. That can then endanger the success of your case altogether.

In sum, your attorney should be experienced enough and successful enough to be able to afford your case. An experienced attorney who has already won numerous nursing home cases understands what your case is about and understands what your needs and concerns are, all while possessing the means to pursue your case from day one all the way to your settlement.

Chapter 12

Now That You Have a Lawyer,

What Should You Expect?

THE FIRST AND PRIMARY REASON for hiring a lawyer was to help you and relieve your anxiety about your loved one's claim. It is now the attorney's responsibility to be there for you and properly prosecute the case.

Once that major step is taken, you can sit back and focus on your loved one's care. Even when your lawyer is working hard behind the scenes for you, there may not be enough progress to require a call every week or even every month with an update. That is because cases move through certain stages as they make their way towards a trial. While very few cases actually go to trial, your attorney has to work thoroughly and aggressively to prepare for trial. This is what causes the case to settle. Sitting back and doing nothing or very little and hoping it will settle is the surest way to end up at trial or an undervalued settlement

If you ever get impatient, need an update, or have a new question, call your lawyer and ask. That is what they are there for.

Returning to the process, in the beginning stages of the case, the first step is for the attorney to gather all the necessary medical records. Depending upon how long your family member has stayed at their nursing home and how many medical providers there have been, that process can take anywhere from one month to several months to complete.

Once the records are obtained, the case will then get reviewed. That will be either an internal review with the attorney or an outside medical review with medical experts, depending on the issues involved in the case. The review process can take anywhere from a few weeks to a few months.

Once the review is completed, you should hear from your lawyer telling you about the results of the review and what the next step is. If your lawyer has decided you have a strong case, the next step will be to file a lawsuit. This can vary in some states where the process is different. Generally speaking, once the lawsuit is filed, the first step is serving papers on the other parties. That is usually about a 30 to 60-day process. Once the nursing home is served with papers, their attorneys will then file their appearance in court.

Once all parties are served and have appeared, the case moves to the next phase, called discovery. The judge will give an extended period of time for discovery, or fact finding. This period is different based on the location of the lawsuit. It may be as short as a few months, or it may be several years. Over the course of the discovery phase, you will likely have to answer some written questions called interrogatories. While you have surely been following the case step by step up to this point, the interrogatories are really your first involvement in the lawsuit. The attorney's office will assist you with answering these questions.

Your next involvement may come on average about 12 to 18 months into the lawsuit. At that point, you may be asked to speak to the lawyers of the other side for a deposition. A deposition is a formal method of taking a witness statement. There will be a court reporter present to transcribe everything the deponent has to say. The attorney calling the deposition is the one who asks the questions. Once your deposition is taken, your active role in the case is minimal until a trial or settlement discussions. The case continues to progress by the taking of other depositions, such as witnesses or medical providers. Your attorney will handle these. There is nothing for you to do at this point. In addition to the depositions, there is also an exchange of records and other documents per each side's request. Again, this is handled by your attorney. As the case progresses closer to a trial date, one of the final stages or steps is the hiring and deposing of the hired experts to support your case. This may be state specific for what cases require experts.

Throughout this entire process, your case can settle at any time. There is no specific timeline for when a settlement may occur. The only event that is on a timeline in your case is the trial, should it be required. If a settlement is not reached in an earlier stage, your case will steadily moved forward toward a jury trial. In that event, your final involvement in the case would be your expected presence at the trial.

However, trials are fairly rare in nursing home cases. They happen less than 5 percent of the time. Most of the cases we see settle prior to that final stage. Just when a settlement will be reached is harder to say. Some cases settle very early on, and some may settle very close to the trial date. It all depends on the evidence, the lawyers, and the individuals involved on both sides.

Many times, in an effort to reach a settlement, your attorney may agree to attend a mediation. Some states require mediation before a case is set for a trial. There are two basic forms of a mediation. Binding and non-binding. A mediation is an informal meeting with an independent judge or mediator that will meet with you, your attorney, and the nursing home's attorney in an effort to settle the case.

A binding mediation is an agreement that if the parties do not agree on a settlement, the mediator will rule on a settlement value, and that is a final settlement on the case. Binding mediations are not very common.

More common, is a non-binding mediation. In this scenario, a mediator is selected, often times a judge or former judge. This mediator sits down with all parties to see if they can come to a settlement agreement without a trial. A lot of nursing home cases will have a mediation scheduled.

That's the overall process your case will go through from day one until the end. It's important to recognize that the above rules are just guidelines. Every case is different, and every state's laws are a little different as well. Some states have a different process in terms of their timing.

If the whole process feels too complicated, don't worry. We always walk our clients through it step by step, preparing them for whatever is ahead. It is our job to keep these events straight so our clients can concentrate on taking care of themselves and their families.

Chapter 13

Never Lose Faith—

That's Why You Have a Lawyer

THROUGHOUT THIS BOOK, we have told some of the stories of those harmed in nursing homes and their families. Although each case was very different, they all had some things in common: the nursing home failed them; the families were desperate for justice; and we were there to provide that justice.

That is what we always do. No matter how difficult the case may be, no matter how tough the nursing home is, we work hard to find a way to get the best results for our clients.

To fully illustrate this, we want to bring up one last story.

One of our cases, several years ago, involved a 75-year-old man with dementia named Charles Reese. Charles' family was unable to safely care for him at home due to his progressing dementia. Charles began wandering out of the home a night, and the family feared for his safety. Therefore, they decided it was time for long-term, skilled nursing care. It was an incredibly hard decision for the family, but they knew they had no choice.

At first, all was seemingly going well. Charles got along well with the staff and other residents in the nursing home. Though, increasingly, he became less and less communicable due to his dementia, he seemed happy when his family visited, and as far as his family could tell, he seemed well taken care of.

Because of his dementia and a previous fall, the nursing home knew he was at risk for another fall. Yet, somehow, he fell anyway. The family got a call one day just a few months after he entered the nursing home saying Charles had fallen, but it wasn't serious, just a little bruise. Unfortunately, this nursing home was quite far from the family, so they were unable to visit very often. Though they made an extra effort after the fall, it was almost a week before they could get to the nursing home. By then, it was clear something was wrong.

The "little bruise" had actually covered half of his face. Even worse, he had clearly lost a significant amount of weight. The family insisted Charles be sent to the hospital, where they discovered he had fractured in his head. He was put on a feeding tube. Although he rallied briefly, his health continued to decline, and after another couple months, Charles Reese died.

His family was beyond devastated, and through all their own feelings of guilt and mourning, they rightly suspected that the nursing home was to blame. Charles never should have fallen, and after he fell, he should have been given better treatment. Charles' family contacted us, and we immediately went to work on their behalf.

As we fought this case, the attorneys representing the nursing home fought back. The nursing home lawyers made every attempt to delay the process, causing months of delays.

This was not surprising, as the nursing home we were going up against was part of a large entity, one that was famous for its stinginess in hiring staff and its aggressiveness in avoiding paying for neglect and abuse that resulted from its understaffing.

These tactics included everything from a failure to respond to important questions on time to a resistance to releasing the documents we needed for Charles' case. While we always try to solve these issues in the simplest and fastest way possible, the nursing home's lawyers were not interested in meeting us halfway. They were trying to freeze us out.

As time passed, and delay was met with more delays, we brought motion after motion to the judge, seeking responses from the defendant in a timely manner. A motion requires a response within a certain period, and if it is not met, the judge on the case can decide on a penalty against the non-responding party.

Still, even after we overcame the nursing home dragging its feet, they made every effort to avoid resolving the strong case we had against them.

Many lawyers do not want to try cases and will attempt to settle a case at any cost. The defendants know that and will bully these lawyers into low settlements by preparing to try the case.

As Charles' trial date was approaching and the nursing home lawyers realized this case was heading towards a jury, the nursing home had no choice but to pay the true value of the case.

This is common. The truth is, in our opinion, nursing homes rarely want to go to trial. A jury will not likely be very sympathetic to a nursing home, as everyone has heard countless stories of nursing home nightmares. In addition, nursing homes would prefer to avoid any negative publicity that a verdict may bring.

Most people already assume that nursing homes are bad, and that's the image that they already have at the start of a trial. That means we, the lawyers of Charles Reese, would enter any trial with a little bit of an advantage. The jury would already be prepared to be against the nursing home.

After all of the delay tactics in Charles' case, we agreed to sit in a mediation to attempt to find a resolution for the family. After eight hours of mediation, Charles Reese's case settled for more than a million dollars.

Charles' children broken down in tears when we told them. It was such a relief, they told us, to finally have some justice for their father, to finally have some recognition of guilt by the nursing home.

"You know," Charles' son, Eric, told us, "it's not even about the money. It's about doing something for Dad. We proved what they did was wrong. I think Dad would be proud of us."

The family told us they had already committed to donating much of the money to charities designed to help the elderly. As is common with our cases, it really is never about the money. It was about being able to speak up against what was wrong, against treatment that had harmed someone they loved. We were able to speak up for them. It allowed them to finally have closure and to move on. That is always the best part of the job for us.

Conclusion

Why We Do What We Do

THE SIMPLE ANSWER to "why we do what we do" is to simply list off the names you've already encountered in this book: Susan Bell and her sons, Heather Reed and her sister Mary, Martina Costa, Jerry Swift, Josephine Sanders, Janet Peters, Naomi Pitt, Michael Kemper, Sarah Jones and her son, Daniel Foresyte, Sylvia Stein, and Charles Reese and his children. We do what we do because someone has to speak up for those who have been harmed and who are unable to speak up for themselves.

Nursing home neglect and abuse is happening every day all across the country. It can and will affect anybody and everybody. We all have parents and grandparents, and you never know who is going to need some type of long-term or short-term care in a nursing home. There is a good chance, at some point in your life, you will have a family member or a friend in this type of situation.

Every day, we hear heartbreaking stories from traumatized families about the poor care their loved ones experienced in a nursing home. These stories are horrific and grossly immoral, and they require justice. No one deserves to be mistreated at the end of their days. And yet, it is happening every single day, in every town and city across this country.

It amazes us that these stories aren't regularly featured on the news. The treatment innocent people suffer through just because they have grown old and sick is appalling to us.

We hope these lawsuits make an impact on the overall care at nursing homes across the country: if not on the overall society and community that we live in, at least to the individual families we represent. Residents and families sometimes feel that nobody believes them when they describe the horrible care, conditions, and abuse that has occurred. When a lawsuit is filed and we prove the neglect that took place, our clients feel justified that something is being done to correct this wrong. Families can now confront those who harmed their loved ones.

In one sense, we think of our work as a public service, because no one else is effectively monitoring nursing homes. Government agencies do the best they can, but unfortunately, it is not enough to stop the abuse and neglect. Neglect and bad care is happening every single day across the country, in almost every nursing home. There is an entire community of elderly and ill people living and suffering in these conditions. We must work together to stop the abuse.

Bad care is not fair, and there is no excuse for it to continue. We believe holding bad acting nursing homes accountable not only saves lives, it is also the right thing to do. We have written this book to do the same. We hope that you have learned something from these pages that can help protect you and your loved ones in the future.

About the Authors

William Pintas

Over the course of his 30-year career, William Pintas has represented more than 10,000 cases, recovering hundreds of millions of dollars for his clients.

Attorney Pintas pursued personal injury law because of his passion for helping injury victims against the powerful and deep-pocketed parties responsible for their injuries. He believes in listening to his clients' unique stories and helping each and every one of them communicate their experiences in court. He never loses sight of how his service can make a difference in his clients' lives.

In 1985, Attorney Pintas founded a firm then known as William G. Pintas & Associates to uphold the laws designed to protect injured victims. Bill Pintas strives to provide every client with strong advocacy and compassionate counsel—the kind they need and deserve after an injury. The firm handles all types of injury cases, including those involving cancer litigation, nursing home and medical negligence, and injuries from pharmaceuticals and medical devices. His firm serves clients in all 50 states.

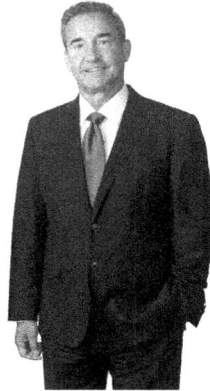

Laura Mullins

Laura Mullins received her bachelor's degree at Syracuse University and graduated John Marshall Law School cum laude with her J.D. She knew early on that she wanted to be a personal injury attorney. Clerking at a personal injury firm in her second year of law school, she immediately connected with the people and the practice. Fighting for the rights of those hurt by the negligence or misconduct of others was—and remains—important to her. She saw the work as valuable and necessary. She enjoyed connecting with all the unique clients and serving them in an important and meaningful way.

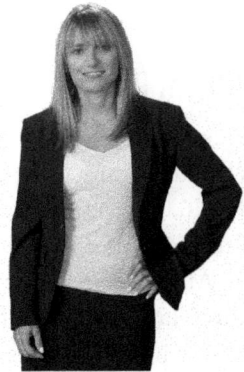

Over the course of her 20-year career, Attorney Mullins has handled thousands of cases. Her compassionate counsel and precise representation has resulted in millions of dollars in successful verdicts and settlements. As a lead attorney at Pintas & Mullins Law Firm, a celebrated law firm based in Chicago and serving clients nationwide, Attorney Mullins is able to provide long-term solutions, compassion, and hope for the future. She is also a Member of the American Association of Justice, the Nursing Home Litigation Group, The Illinois Trials Lawyers Association, and the Decalogue Society.

Attorney Mullins takes a unique approach to personal injury representation. She truly views herself as a counselor, contributing to her clients' overall wellbeing. She is a listener and a doer; she hears her clients' concerns and does everything in her power to fight for her clients. Her clients know that they are not alone; they are in experienced hands.

Attorney Mullins specializes in nursing home injuries.

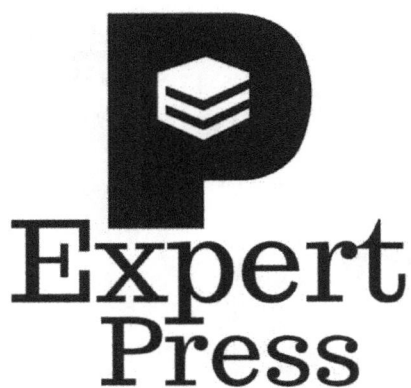

www.ingramcontent.com/pod-product-compliance
Lightning Source LLC
Chambersburg PA
CBHW071606200326
41519CB00021BB/6885